The No BS Way: Lose Weight, Get Real Results

By Alex Ryder

Table of Contents

Introduction

This isn't your typical fitness book full of empty promises. If you're tired of being lied to about what it takes to lose weight and get fit, you've come to the right place. In this book, we're cutting through the noise, throwing out the gimmicks, and focusing on the **TRUTH**.

For too long, fitness gurus have sold you fantasies—telling you what you want to hear instead of what actually works. They market quick-fix solutions that don't last. Diet pills, detox teas, and fad diets might promise the world, but in the end, they leave you frustrated and feeling like a failure. **Why?** Because they ignore the fundamentals, giving you temporary results at best or no results at all.

The truth is, **the method of losing weight is extremely simple**—you need to eat less, move more, and be consistent. But here's the catch: **doing it is extremely hard**. It takes dedication, discipline, and a willingness to stick with it when things get tough. There's no secret, no shortcut, and no magic pill that can replace those basics.

This book is different. We're not going to promise you **instant results**—because those don't last. What we will give you is the blueprint to achieve **the real, lasting results** you've been chasing. You won't see overnight changes, but you will see **the results that actually matter**—results you can maintain for the rest of your life. No gimmicks, no fluff, just straight-up truth.

Why Listen to Me?

You might be wondering—**who am I, and why should you listen to me?** I'm not a celebrity trainer, I don't have a reality TV show, and I'm not here to sell you a miracle diet. I'm just an ordinary guy with a passion for bodybuilding that started when I was 14 years old. I've been there, done that, and like you, I've faced every challenge that comes with the fitness journey.

I've gone through the ups and downs of building muscle and losing fat. I've spent years trying different diets, countless hours in the gym, and wasted time on things that didn't work. But what's important to understand is that **I've been through the struggles you're facing right now**. I know what it's like to feel frustrated when you're not seeing results, when you're bombarded by misleading information, or when you just don't know where to start.

For me, the hardest part was **losing the weight**. I was constantly searching for shortcuts, trying quick fixes that promised fast results—only to be disappointed over and over again. I didn't get the abs I wanted until I accepted the truth: there is no magic pill, no fancy workout routine, no secret formula. **It took dedication, consistency, and a willingness to do things the right way.**

I also know what it's like to be overwhelmed by all the conflicting advice out there—some telling you to eat carbs, others saying to avoid them; some trainers saying to lift heavy, others saying to focus on cardio. It's exhausting. And after years of trial and error, I finally cut through the noise and figured out what really works.

I'm not here to offer quick fixes or empty promises. **What I'm offering is a practical, real-world approach** to fitness—an approach based on **common sense**, **discipline**, and the **principles** that actually lead to lasting results. I've made the mistakes so you don't have to.

This book is not filled with complicated jargon or unrealistic expectations. It's based on my experience, real-world strategies, and proven methods that have worked for me and for others who were in the same boat. I'm not telling you what you want to hear; I'm telling you what you need to hear.

If you're tired of the lies, the false promises, and the confusing information that's out there, then I'm here to give you the **truth**, without the fluff. I know the pain, frustration, and self-doubt you've probably felt. I've been there. But I've also found the way out. And I'm here to guide you through it.

The Problem

The fitness industry is built on selling dreams. You see it everywhere—perfectly toned bodies on Instagram, 30-day transformation challenges, and "miracle" weight loss products that claim to melt fat overnight. But here's the problem: most of these methods are either ineffective, unsustainable, or downright lies.

And it's not just the fitness industry. The **pharmaceutical industry**, the **diet industry**, and even **self-help gurus** operate in the same way. They thrive on selling **quick fixes** to long-term problems. Whether it's a diet pill, a detox tea, or a secret formula for success, these industries know that giving you **temporary results**—or no results at all—keeps you coming back. It's all designed to create a **cycle of hope and failure**.

Here's how it works: they promise you an easy solution, something that seems too good to be true—and it usually is. You get excited, you try it, and maybe you even see some short-term results. But those results never last, because the solution isn't addressing the root problem. So, you end up right back where you started, frustrated and feeling like you failed. And what's the first thing you do? You look for the next quick fix. And the cycle repeats.

Why do they do this? Because it's profitable. The goal is not to actually fix your problem—it's to keep you **coming back and spending your hard-earned money**. If they solved your issue once and for all, they'd lose you as a customer. So instead, they give you just enough hope to keep you hooked, knowing full well you'll be back when their solution doesn't deliver in the long term.

This is why the fitness industry thrives on new trends, diets, and "breakthrough" products. They're not selling you a path to lasting results; they're selling you an illusion. And that illusion costs you time, money, and your sanity.

The Truth

But here's the truth: **there are no shortcuts**. Real results require effort, consistency, and a focus on the fundamentals. If you want to lose weight and keep it off, you need to **eat less than you burn, train effectively, and rest properly**. It's simple, but not always easy. And that's exactly what the fitness and diet industries don't want you to realize—because if you understood how simple it actually is, you wouldn't need their endless stream of products, diets, and programs.

The No BS Way

So, how do we fix this? Enter the **No BS Way**. This isn't your typical fitness approach, and this certainly isn't another fad diet or quick-fix solution. In this book, we're not selling dreams or offering you a "magic bullet." Instead, we're giving you an approach that strips away all the nonsense and focuses on what actually works.

Forget the overcomplicated diets, the miracle weight loss pills, or the unrealistic transformation challenges. We're going back to basics. We're focusing on what works, and only what works.

The **No BS Way** is simple and straightforward:

1. **Eating in a calorie deficit**: To lose fat, you need to consume fewer calories than you burn. Period. No need for counting every calorie to the last detail—just a simple understanding of how much you're consuming and how much you need to burn.

2. **Strength training to build muscle and burn fat**: Strength training is the foundation of any fat loss journey. By building muscle, you increase your metabolism, which means you burn more calories at rest. It's the key to getting lean and strong.

3. **Cardio for heart health and fat loss**: Cardio is important, but it's not the main way to lose fat. It's about using cardio wisely to supplement your strength training, keep your heart healthy, and burn additional calories.

4. **Discipline to stay consistent**: The hardest part of any fitness journey is discipline. The No BS Way requires you to stay consistent, even when motivation fades. It's about making the right choice every day, even when it's tough, because you know it's the right thing to do for your goals.

Here's the hard truth—this book won't give you results if you don't give yourself permission to succeed. There's no magic pill, no secret formula, and no quick fix. The only thing standing between you and results is your own **discipline**. That's the truth. If you're still waiting for some easy solution, or if you're just looking for another reason to avoid doing the work, this book isn't for you.

Aren't you tired of complaining that it's not working? Tired of blaming genetics, or saying, "I don't have time," or "It's just too hard"? Those are excuses, and excuses won't get you results. The truth is, we all have the same 24 hours in a day, and we all face challenges. The difference between those who succeed and those who don't is how they respond to those challenges.

The **No BS Way** is about taking full responsibility for your progress. If you keep messing around and thinking you can "try" your way into fitness, you'll end up exactly where you are now—frustrated, stuck, and nowhere near your goals. It's not about motivation or willpower alone; it's about **discipline**. The kind of discipline that sticks when motivation fades.

And here's the real kicker—you don't have to give up pizza or beer to get fit. What you need to do is stop putting them on a pedestal like they're the only choices that make life enjoyable. Sure, after a long day, it's tempting to grab a pizza and wash it down with five beers, but that's not the only way to unwind or reward yourself. The decision to take care of your body doesn't mean you'll never enjoy those foods again. It just means you'll learn how to enjoy them in moderation.

For this to work, you won't need to say goodbye to the things you love. You'll just need to **kick them down from their pedestal** and stop letting them dictate your health or your energy levels. Instead of ordering a pizza when you're tired and throwing back beers to relax, you can choose to make a quick, easy, and delicious healthy meal—and pair it with sparkling water or a low-calorie drink. It's about finding balance and making choices that leave you feeling good in the long run, not guilty.

This book gives you the tools, the knowledge, and the guidance. But **you have to bring the commitment**. You have to stop screwing around and decide to make it happen. There's no one else to blame, and no excuses left. If you're tired of playing games and ready to take real action, then let's get started.

What You'll Learn

Here's what you can expect from this book:

- **The TRUTH About Weight Loss**: We'll tear down the myths and lies that have kept you stuck in a cycle of frustration. You'll learn the real, unfiltered truth about what it takes to shed fat and keep it off—for good. Spoiler alert: it's not as complicated as you've been led to believe.

- **The No BS Diet**: No more restrictive fad diets or endless calorie counting. I'll teach you how to eat for weight loss in a way that's sustainable and doesn't make you miserable. You'll learn how to enjoy your food without guilt and still hit your goals.

- **Workout Plans**: You'll get gym routines that maximize fat loss while building strength and muscle. No fluff, no wasting hours in the gym—just the most efficient way to get the body you want. Strength training will be your best friend, and I'll show you why.

- **Recovery**: We'll dive into the often-overlooked piece of the puzzle—rest, recovery, and stress management. You'll learn why these are just as important as your workouts and diet, and how to make sure you're recovering properly to avoid burnout and injury.

- **Staying Consistent**: Discipline is what separates success from failure. You'll learn how to build lasting habits that keep you on track even when life throws curveballs. This section will arm you with the strategies to stay consistent, even when motivation fades.

Each chapter is designed to give you the essential information you need—without overcomplicating things. My goal is for you to finish this book feeling confident, equipped, and ready to take control of your fitness journey, knowing exactly what steps to take and why.

Why This Works

This approach isn't based on trendy diets or the latest fitness fads. It's grounded in science and backed by real-world results. I've seen it work time and time again—not just in my own life, but with countless others who, like you, were tired of being misled by the fitness industry's false promises.

The reason it works is simple: it's rooted in reality. We're focusing on methods you can sustain for the long haul, not just for the next 30 days or until your motivation fades. This isn't about a quick fix that gives you short-term results only to leave you back where you started once you stop some impossible routine. It's about building a lifestyle that lasts.

These principles don't rely on gimmicks or temporary solutions. They're about creating habits that stick, balancing fitness with real life, and staying consistent without obsessing over every detail. And I promise you—this works. It's realistic, it's sustainable, and it's been proven to get results time and time again.

Call to Action

If you're tired of chasing quick fixes and ready to commit to a plan that actually works, you've come to the right place. The No BS Way is your roadmap to lasting success—but remember, there are no shortcuts. What you'll need is commitment, consistency, and the willingness to embrace the process, even when it's challenging.

Now, you have two choices. You can close this book, keep doing what you've always done, and stay stuck in the same cycle of frustration, disappointment, and feeling like you're not enough. Or, you can make the decision right now to step up, take control, and finally get the results you've always wanted.

This is the start of something real. If you're ready to stop making excuses and start putting in the work, let's get to it. The results are waiting for you. It's time to make them happen.

Chapter 1: The TRUTH About Weight Loss

Let's get one thing straight—weight loss doesn't have to be complicated, but it's not always as easy as people make it seem either.

You've heard it all before: "Eat less, move more, and you'll lose weight." But if it's that simple, why do so many people fail? It's because, in reality, it's not about being complex—it's about sticking with it. The reason most people don't see results isn't because the method doesn't work, but because they don't give it enough time or consistency. You try something for two days, see no significant change, and immediately give up, thinking it's not working.

But here's the truth—results take time. **Weight loss is a marathon, not a sprint.** And if you think you'll see drastic changes in a matter of days, you're setting yourself up for failure. The problem is, we live in a world of instant gratification, and when we don't see quick results, we start doubting ourselves and the process.

So, what happens next? You quit. Or worse—you complicate things. You start thinking maybe you're not doing the right diet, or you need a more complex workout plan, or that you need to buy some overpriced supplement that promises to speed things up. But the more you complicate it, the harder it gets. The simple truths become buried under layers of confusion. And eventually, you just feel mentally drained, stuck, and discouraged.

The mental toll is real. The stress of trying to fit into a new routine or stick with a diet that's unsustainable can wear you out. And this is why most people fail. It's not the plan—it's the lack of patience, the lack of consistency, and the lack of belief that you can actually stick with it long enough to see results.

So, what's the solution? It's simple. **Stop overcomplicating it.** Stop expecting overnight success. Stop making excuses when the scale doesn't move in two days. Instead, focus on the fundamentals—the stuff that works. And here's the best part: You don't need to reinvent the wheel.

In this chapter, I'm going to strip away the myths and show you how easy weight loss really can be when you approach it with the right mindset and the right strategy. You'll learn why the key to success isn't about extreme diets or complicated workout plans—it's about doing the right things consistently, day after day.

The truth is, weight loss is less about willpower and more about **discipline**. It's not about how much you push yourself in a single workout; it's about making those small, consistent choices every day that add up to real results.

Are you ready to get real and stop the cycle of frustration? Let's dive in.

Weight Loss Is Simple, But Not Easy

Let's start with the most important fact: weight loss is simple, but it's not easy.

You don't need a complex formula or an expensive supplement to lose weight. In fact, the fundamentals of weight loss are very straightforward. At its core, it's about two things: consuming fewer calories than you burn and staying consistent.

But here's the catch—just because something is simple doesn't mean it's easy. If it were that easy, everyone would be fit and lean, right? The reason why so many people struggle with weight loss isn't because the concept is difficult—it's because we overcomplicate things and let our minds get in the way.

We live in a world of shortcuts. The fitness industry has conditioned us to believe that we can have quick results, and that if we don't see them within days, we must be doing something wrong. We start second-guessing the method, jumping from diet to diet, trying new workouts, buying pills, or following the latest trend that promises a fast fix.

But let me be clear: there's no magic trick—just a simple formula. You don't need to count every calorie, follow every restriction, or do extreme workouts. All you need to do is focus on the basics and remain patient.

The Real Struggle: Consistency Over Perfection

The biggest issue most people face is not sticking to the plan. We've all been there: you start a diet or a new workout plan, and you're feeling great for the first few days, but after a couple of days—or even a couple of hours—you hit a bump. You don't see the results you were expecting. Maybe you don't see a change on the scale, or you still feel tired after your workouts. And that's when the doubts start creeping in.

"Is this really working?"

"I'm eating healthy, but the weight isn't coming off fast enough."

"I don't have time for this; I'll just have that pizza tonight."

This mindset is what trips people up, and it's why they fail. Results take time, and it's the slow and steady progress that leads to long-lasting success. If you expect to see a complete transformation overnight or even within a week, you'll always feel like you're falling short.

The truth is, weight loss is a marathon, not a sprint. It's about making those small, consistent decisions every day. Whether you're choosing a healthy meal over fast food, sticking to your workout routine, or getting enough sleep, these daily choices add up over time. They may not seem like much in the moment, but they make all the difference in the long run.

Understanding the Basics

Let's break down the simplicity of it all:

Calories In vs. Calories Out

To lose weight, you need to consume fewer calories than you burn. It's that simple.

Imagine your body is like a car. It needs fuel to run—just like a car needs gas to drive. Every time you eat, you're putting fuel (calories) into your body. Your body, like a car engine, burns fuel to keep everything running smoothly: breathing, digestion, movement—everything you do requires energy.

Now, just like a car, your body needs a specific amount of fuel each day to operate. This is where **calories in and calories out** come into play:

- **Calories In**: This is the food you eat, the fuel you're putting into your body. Every meal, every snack, every drink you have adds fuel to your "tank."

- **Calories Out**: This is the energy your body uses to function. Even when you're sitting still, your body is burning calories to keep your heart beating, your lungs working, and your organs functioning. The more you move—whether it's exercising, walking, or even fidgeting—the more fuel your body burns.

Just like your car, if you put too much fuel in (eat too many calories) and don't burn it off, your body stores the excess as fat. But if you put in less fuel (eat fewer calories) than you need, your body burns its own fat stores for energy, and that's how weight loss happens.

The basic rule is simple: **If you burn more calories than you consume, you'll lose weight. If you consume more than you burn, you'll gain weight.**

Movement: The Cherry on Top

Exercise is the cherry on top. While exercise isn't absolutely necessary for weight loss, it speeds up the process and makes it more sustainable. Strength training builds muscle, which increases your metabolism and helps burn more calories even while you're resting. Cardio improves your heart health and burns additional calories, but you don't need to spend hours doing it. Even small amounts of movement can help.

Consistency: The Key to Success

Here's where most people fall off track: it's not about doing something perfectly once or twice; it's about doing the right things **consistently**. It's about showing up every day, even when you don't feel like it. Whether it's choosing a healthier snack, hitting the gym, or getting an extra hour of sleep, these small, daily actions add up over time and build momentum.

Mindset: Embrace the Journey

The mental game is the hardest part of weight loss. It's easy to get frustrated when results don't come as quickly as you want. But the key is to **embrace the journey**, not just the destination. Weight loss is a process—it will take time, but with the right mindset, you can stay consistent and keep moving forward.

Why People Fail

So, if weight loss is simple, why do so many people fail?

There are several reasons why people struggle to see results, and it's rarely because they don't "know" what to do. In fact, most people already know the basics: eat less, move more. But the real issue is that **they don't follow through** or they **overcomplicate the process**.

Here's why people often fail:

1. They don't follow the diet consistently

The most common reason people fail is that they don't stick to their diet plan long enough. They may follow it for a few days, but the moment they hit a roadblock or don't see instant results, they go off course. Whether it's indulging in extra portions, skipping workouts, or eating something "off-plan," inconsistency is the number one killer of progress. Weight loss doesn't happen overnight, and expecting quick results often leads to frustration and giving up too soon.

2. They eat too many calories, even while exercising

Here's where the problem lies: you can run or work out as much as you want, but if you're eating more calories than you burn, the weight won't come off. People often fall into the trap of thinking they can eat whatever they want because they exercise. However, it's easy to underestimate how many calories you're consuming, especially with "healthy" snacks, or portions that are larger than you realize. If your body is getting more fuel (calories) than it needs, it will store the excess as fat, no matter how much you exercise.

3. They follow misleading or outdated advice

Here's another reason people get stuck: they follow outdated or ridiculous rules that don't actually help with weight loss. Things like "don't eat white bread," "cut out carbs," or "avoid sugar at all costs." While those things may sound helpful, they can actually lead to confusion and frustration. The truth is, it's not about avoiding one type of food or another—it's about understanding the bigger picture of how your body works and creating a plan that fits your lifestyle.

4. They fall for quick fixes or fad diets

We live in a world filled with false promises: detox diets, miracle pills, and extreme meal plans that guarantee fast results. But here's the hard truth: there is no magic bullet for weight loss. Quick fixes may lead to short-term results, but they aren't sustainable in the long run. People who chase fad diets often end up stuck in a cycle of yo-yo dieting, gaining back the weight they lose, and then some.

5. They overcomplicate the process

Weight loss doesn't need to be complicated, but people often make it harder than it needs to be. They count every calorie, micromanage every meal, and overthink every workout. They spend hours reading the latest fitness articles or trying to figure out the "perfect" routine. But this approach only leads to burnout. Instead of focusing on a sustainable lifestyle, they burn out trying to follow complex plans. The result? They give up, discouraged, and confused about what went wrong.

6. They expect instant results

Here's a major hurdle: people expect to see results quickly and when they don't, they quit. If you're expecting to drop 10 pounds in a week or see visible abs in just a few days, you're setting yourself up for failure. Weight loss is a gradual process. If you're looking for instant results, you're going to feel like you're failing, even if you're making progress. This expectation of immediate change can be mentally exhausting, leading to feelings of disappointment and discouragement.

Overcoming These Challenges

The key to overcoming these obstacles is **simple consistency**. Weight loss happens when you:

- **Stick to your diet plan** long enough to see results.
- **Track your calories** accurately to ensure you're in a deficit (without obsessing over every little thing).
- **Cut out the myths** (such as avoiding specific foods like white bread) and focus on eating a balanced, sustainable diet.
- **Forget about quick fixes** and focus on long-term changes.
- **Simplify the process** rather than overcomplicating it.

If you're still clinging to old myths or expecting to drop pounds overnight, you're setting yourself up for failure. But if you're ready to accept that weight loss is a process and that it takes time, then you're on the right track.

Success comes when you **embrace consistency, forget the shortcuts, and stay patient**. When you focus on real, sustainable changes and stop falling for the next big trend or quick-fix diet, that's when the magic happens.

Overcoming These Challenges: Fuel and Patience

The key takeaway here is that **weight loss is like fueling your car**: it's not about adding the fuel and seeing the car speed off right away. You fill the tank, and over time, your body starts to use the fuel it needs. Similarly, when you eat the right amount of calories for weight loss and burn through your daily activities, the process takes time.

Stay consistent. Trust the process. Don't expect overnight success.

Just like a car needs time to burn fuel and travel the distance, your body needs time to burn fat and transform. You wouldn't expect your car to go from zero to sixty the second you add fuel, so don't expect to see drastic changes in your body overnight either.

Here's the real truth: the most successful people are the ones who **show up every day**, even when the results aren't immediate. It's the small, consistent efforts over time that add up to lasting transformation.

Patience is key. Give your body the time it needs to do its work. And while you're at it, stay focused on the bigger picture—remember, weight loss isn't a sprint; it's a marathon. Just as your car keeps moving forward with every drop of fuel, your body will keep burning fat and getting leaner with every healthy choice you make.

Debunking the Myths

When it comes to weight loss, the amount of misinformation out there is overwhelming. It seems like every time you open a magazine, scroll through social media, or tune into a fitness podcast, there's a new "miracle" diet or workout routine being sold to you. From fad diets to extreme exercise programs, the fitness industry is notorious for creating confusion and making things seem much harder than they need to be.

So, why do we fall for these myths?
It's simple: people are desperate for quick results. We want to lose weight fast, without realizing that long-term success requires patience, consistency, and, most importantly, a **scientific understanding** of how our bodies work.

The truth is, while these myths might sound convincing or even have some element of truth, they are not the key to sustainable weight loss. In fact, they often create more problems than they solve, leading to frustration, confusion, and sometimes even weight gain.

This chapter will expose the most common myths surrounding weight loss and help you understand why they're not just wrong but harmful to your progress. By breaking down these misconceptions, we'll get to the root of why **weight loss is simple, but it's not easy.**

In the following pages, I'll debunk the top myths you've likely heard a thousand times, separating fact from fiction, and giving you the clarity you need to succeed. From the belief that carbs are the enemy to the idea that you can target fat loss in specific areas, you'll see why these myths not only mislead you but actually get in the way of your success.

Get ready to cut through the noise and learn the truth about weight loss—because it's time to stop believing in nonsense and start seeing real results.

Myth #1: "Extreme Dieting is the Fastest Way to Lose Weight"

One of the most prevalent myths surrounding weight loss is the belief that extreme dieting is the fastest way to shed pounds. This myth promises rapid results, but what it doesn't tell you is that the cost to your health and long-term well-being is often far greater than the temporary weight loss.

The truth is, extreme diets that cut out entire food groups or drastically reduce calories can lead to dangerous side effects. When you cut out essential vitamins, minerals, and nutrients, your body doesn't just lose fat; it also loses the fuel it needs to function properly. This can result in hormonal imbalances, fatigue, and a feeling of total exhaustion.

The Toll of Extreme Dieting

To illustrate the dangers of extreme diets, look at professional athletes who engage in drastic weight cuts to meet weight classes for competitions. Fighters, for example, often undergo severe dehydration and food restriction in the days leading up to a fight, only to rehydrate and replenish themselves hours before stepping into the ring. The day before the fight, they're often exhausted, miserable, and feeling completely drained—both physically and mentally.

Similarly, bodybuilders who are preparing for a competition often go through weeks or even months of extreme dieting, cutting carbohydrates and fat to the bare minimum. The day of the competition, they may look shredded and lean, but they feel awful—low energy, mentally foggy, and completely depleted.

These extreme measures aren't just uncomfortable; they're dangerous. When you deprive your body of essential nutrients, your hormones can become unbalanced, leading to low energy, mood swings, and potentially long-term damage to your metabolism. This is why extreme diets should never be the go-to solution for anyone seeking sustainable weight loss.

Takeaway:
Extreme dieting may give you quick results, but it often comes with unwanted side effects like nutrient deficiencies, hormonal imbalances, and loss of muscle mass. Focus on sustainable, balanced changes that nourish your body and promote healthy fat loss over time. The key to lasting results isn't drastic restrictions—it's consistency, moderation, and taking care of your body along the way.

Myth #2: "Carbs Make You Fat"

Ah, the infamous "carbs make you fat" myth. This one is everywhere. It's plastered across social media, perpetuated by fad diets, and even recommended by people who should know better. But let's set the record straight—carbohydrates **don't make you fat**. In fact, carbs are an essential part of a healthy diet and are a critical fuel source for your body. The real issue is **overeating** and **calorie imbalance**, not carbs themselves.

Carbs: The Body's Preferred Fuel

Your body breaks down carbohydrates into glucose, which it uses as its primary source of energy. Without carbs, your body would struggle to perform even basic functions like walking, breathing, or thinking. If you've ever felt sluggish or mentally foggy after skipping carbs, you know exactly how important they are for keeping your body and brain running efficiently.

But, here's the thing: while carbs are important, it's still possible to overeat them. Just like with protein or fat, if you eat **more calories from carbs than your body needs**, you'll gain weight. It's not carbs themselves that lead to weight gain—it's the total number of calories you consume in relation to the number you burn.

The Low-Carb Diet Fad

Low-carb diets, like keto, have gained a lot of attention in recent years, but they promote the idea that you can lose weight by drastically cutting carbs. What they don't mention is that this method isn't sustainable for most people in the long term. You may lose weight quickly in the beginning, but that's often because you're drastically reducing calories by cutting out foods like bread, pasta, and rice, not because you've found the magical secret to weight loss.

In the end, cutting carbs can lead to a lack of essential nutrients. Whole grains, fruits, and vegetables—rich in fiber, vitamins, and minerals—are crucial for overall health. So, if you're cutting carbs, you're likely cutting out much-needed nutrients.

Why the "Carbs Make You Fat" Myth is Simply Untrue

When it comes down to it, weight gain or loss has to do with calories, not a specific food group. If you're eating more calories than your body needs, whether from carbs, fat, or protein, you will gain weight. But if you're eating the right amount of calories for your body and staying active, carbs are not your enemy.

So the next time someone says carbs make you fat, just shake your head and keep enjoying that piece of whole grain toast or those sweet potatoes. Carbs are your friend, not your foe.

Takeaway:
Carbs aren't the enemy! They're an essential energy source for your body. The key is choosing the right carbs—whole grains, fruits, and veggies—over processed sugars and refined grains. Balance is what matters. Eat carbs in moderation, and focus on your total calorie intake and nutrient quality, not just avoiding them entirely.

Myth #3: "Cardio Is the Only Way to Lose Weight"

Another common myth that needs to be addressed is the idea that cardio is the only way to lose weight. This myth is so widespread that people believe if they're not running on a treadmill or cycling for hours, they're not going to lose any weight. In reality, while cardio can certainly help burn calories, it's not the be-all and end-all of weight loss.

The Truth:

When it comes to weight loss, cardio is just one part of the equation. Yes, it burns calories, but it's not the only way to create a caloric deficit. The most important factor for weight loss is how many calories you're consuming versus how many you're burning.

That means, whether you're doing strength training, high-intensity interval training (HIIT), or even walking, as long as you're burning more calories than you consume, you'll be losing weight.

But let's not forget that strength training has its own advantages when it comes to weight loss. It builds muscle, and muscle burns more calories even while you're at rest. So, while cardio burns calories during the workout, strength training helps boost your metabolism so you burn more calories over time, even when you're not working out.

Why It's a Myth:

The misconception that cardio is the only way to lose weight comes from the fact that people often think of "weight loss" as just fat loss, and cardio can help speed up the process. But it's much more than just burning calories during exercise—it's about long-term changes to your body composition and metabolism.

Strength training is a great way to build muscle, and muscle mass will help you burn more calories throughout the day. Plus, it makes you stronger and improves overall body function, including the health of your heart—because yes, your heart is a muscle, too!

So, don't be fooled into thinking that you need to run for hours to lose weight. While cardio can be part of the equation, strength training and other forms of exercise are just as important for reaching your goals.

Takeaway:
Cardio is great for heart health and calorie burning, but it's not the only route to weight loss. Strength training builds muscle, which boosts your metabolism and helps you burn more calories at rest. Don't underestimate the rush of building muscle—it not only transforms your body but also gives you a long-term fat-burning engine. A balanced approach—incorporating both cardio and resistance training—will give you the best results in the long run.

Myth #4: "Fat-Free or Low-Fat Foods Are Always Healthier"

The "fat-free" craze has been around for decades, with many people believing that anything labeled as "fat-free" or "low-fat" must automatically be the healthier option. In fact, entire aisles in grocery stores are dedicated to "light" or "fat-free" versions of products, from cookies to ice cream. The idea is that if fat is the villain, cutting it out of your diet must be the solution to weight loss and overall health, right? Well, not exactly.

The Truth:

Not all fats are bad. In fact, fats are a crucial part of a balanced diet and serve several important functions in the body. Fat aids in the absorption of fat-soluble vitamins (A, D, E, and K), supports hormone production, and plays a vital role in maintaining healthy skin, hair, and cell function. It also helps regulate digestion by allowing the body to properly break down and absorb nutrients from food.

So why is the fat-free myth misleading? In many cases, when food manufacturers remove fat from a product, they replace it with sugar, refined carbs, or other artificial ingredients to maintain flavor or texture. This can actually make the food less healthy and more calorie-dense in other ways.

The Low-Fat Trap:

Take "fat-free" yogurt, for example. While the fat content may be low, the sugar content in some fat-free yogurts is sky-high. This can cause insulin spikes, contribute to cravings, and even promote fat storage—making it counterproductive to weight loss. Fat-free processed snacks and baked goods might be lower in fat, but they're often higher in carbs, sugars, and artificial additives, all of which can add up to more calories and weight gain if consumed in excess.

The problem with this myth is that it leads people to believe that eating "low-fat" or "fat-free" foods is a free pass to overeat without worrying about calories. But calories matter. You can still gain weight eating "fat-free" products if you're consuming too many calories from other sources, like sugar and carbs.

Good Fats vs. Bad Fats:

Not all fats are created equal, and it's important to distinguish between good and bad fats. Unhealthy fats—like trans fats and excessive saturated fats—can negatively affect your cholesterol levels, increase inflammation, and raise your risk of heart disease. These types of fats are often found in processed, fried, and packaged foods.

On the other hand, healthy fats, such as monounsaturated and polyunsaturated fats, are essential for overall health. They help to lower bad cholesterol (LDL), reduce inflammation, and support heart health. Healthy fats can be found in foods like avocados, nuts, seeds, olive oil, and fatty fish like salmon.

The Real Focus:

Instead of focusing solely on fat content, aim to choose whole, nutrient-dense foods that provide healthy fats. Foods like avocados, nuts, seeds, olive oil, and fatty fish (like salmon) are excellent sources of good fats that support your overall health and metabolism.

When looking at food labels, instead of just focusing on whether something is "low-fat," check the ingredient list for added sugars and other hidden calories. Look at the full picture of the food's nutritional profile, not just one isolated nutrient like fat.

Why It's a Myth:

Not all fats are created equal. While unhealthy trans fats and excessive saturated fats can harm your health by raising cholesterol and causing other issues, healthy fats are essential for optimal function. Fat is vital for digestion, vitamin absorption, hormone regulation, and maintaining healthy cells. Fat-free or low-fat foods might seem like a better choice on the surface, but often they come with a host of unwanted ingredients that can derail your health and weight loss goals.

So, rather than focusing on avoiding fat altogether, focus on choosing healthy, whole foods with balanced fat content. Quality matters far more than fat content alone.

Takeaway:
Not all fats are bad. Healthy fats play a vital role in your body, from hormone regulation to aiding digestion. Fat-free or low-fat foods may seem like the healthier option, but many are packed with sugar or other additives. Focus on eating nutrient-dense, whole foods, and don't be afraid of incorporating good fats into your diet.

Myth #5: "You Can Target Fat Loss in Specific Areas"

The desire to lose fat in specific areas of the body is a common goal, but unfortunately, it's a myth that has been perpetuated for years. Many people believe that doing hundreds of crunches will give them a flat belly, or endless squats will burn fat from their thighs and butt. The concept is often called **spot reduction**—the idea that you can burn fat in a specific area of your body by focusing exercise on that area. But here's the truth: spot reduction simply doesn't work.

The Truth:

When you lose fat, your body decides where the fat comes from. You can't dictate which part of your body burns fat first, just like you can't control where the water level drops when you pour it out of a glass. Fat loss is a whole-body process, and it's determined by genetics, body composition, and overall calorie deficit—not by targeting specific areas with exercises.

The Glass of Water Analogy:

Think of your body like a glass of water. Imagine you want to lower the water level in the glass. You can't just target the top part of the water and expect it to go down while leaving the rest untouched. If you pour out some water, the entire level drops evenly.

Similarly, when you exercise or eat to lose fat, your body burns fat from all areas, not just from the part you're working on. Whether you're doing ab exercises or leg lifts, you're not specifically targeting fat loss in those areas. Your body decides where fat will be lost, and it's a gradual, overall process.

Why It's a Myth:

Fat cells are stored all over your body, and there's no way to control which fat cells are used first. While exercises like crunches and leg raises will help tone and strengthen muscles in a specific area, they won't magically "melt" the fat covering those muscles. To lose fat from a specific area, you need to lose fat from your entire body, and that requires creating a calorie deficit through diet and exercise.

A great analogy is the water glass: you can't pour water from just one part of the glass without lowering the level in the whole thing. In the same way, fat loss happens uniformly across your body. The more consistent you are with your caloric deficit, the more fat your body will burn overall, including the stubborn spots.

The Reality of Fat Loss:

The only way to reveal your abs, trim down your thighs, or lean out your arms is by reducing your overall body fat. This is done through a combination of proper diet (calorie deficit) and exercise (strength training and cardio). While you can build and define muscles in specific areas (like doing core exercises to strengthen your abs), those muscles won't show if they're hidden under layers of fat.

You might tone your muscles with targeted exercises, but fat loss will occur all over your body as your body burns fat for energy, and how much fat you lose from specific areas depends on your genetics and body composition.

The Key:

Instead of wasting energy trying to "target" fat in specific areas, focus on overall fat loss through consistent cardio, strength training, and proper nutrition. As you lose fat, you'll eventually reveal the muscle definition you've been working for. Be patient—it's a whole-body process, and no matter how much you work one area, you can't skip the rest.

Myth #6: "You Have to Skip Meals to Lose Weight"

Skipping meals might seem like a quick fix for weight loss, especially if you're trying to shed pounds fast. The logic often sounds like this: "If I don't eat, I'll burn fat faster." However, this myth is not only misleading—it can also work against your weight loss goals and leave you feeling sluggish or overeating later on.

The Reality:

Skipping meals can actually slow down your metabolism and hinder your ability to lose weight. When you don't eat regularly, your body goes into "starvation mode," where your metabolism slows down to preserve energy. As a result, when you finally do eat, your body tends to store the food as fat because it's trying to hold onto whatever calories it can.

Additionally, skipping meals can leave you feeling more fatigued, irritable, and deprived. This can make it harder to stay on track with healthy eating and often leads to overeating when you finally do get a chance to eat, undoing any progress made earlier in the day.

Balanced Meals = Steady Progress:

The key to successful weight loss is consistency. Eating smaller, balanced meals throughout the day helps keep your metabolism active and your energy levels stable. Your body needs a regular intake of nutrients to function properly. By eating at regular intervals, you provide your body with a steady supply of fuel, which keeps your metabolism humming and prevents the temptation to overeat later on.

Skipping meals, especially for extended periods, can also impact your blood sugar levels, leading to low energy, mood swings, and cravings for unhealthy foods. A steady intake of food ensures you stay fueled, avoid crashes, and make better choices when it comes to portion sizes.

The Role of Fasting:

Now, let's be clear—while skipping meals is not the best strategy, **fasting** (on a controlled basis) can have some benefits. Fasting isn't about depriving your body or skipping meals all the time—it's about giving your body a break from constant digestion, which can be beneficial for fat loss and hormone regulation.

For example, intermittent fasting (such as the 16:8 method, where you eat within an 8-hour window and fast for 16 hours) is popular among some fitness enthusiasts and has shown some potential benefits for fat loss. **Studies** have found that fasting for short periods can help increase levels of Human Growth Hormone (HGH), which is important for muscle preservation and fat loss. One recent study found that HGH levels increased five-fold after a 24-hour fast in a group of 47 participants.

However, it's important to note that **fasting** is not the same as **skipping meals** in the traditional sense. Fasting involves planned and controlled periods of no eating, while skipping meals is often random and inconsistent. When done right, fasting can help with fat loss, but it's not the secret to weight loss on its own.

The Takeaway:

To lose weight in a healthy, sustainable way, skip the idea of skipping meals. Instead, aim to fuel your body with regular, balanced meals throughout the day, and maintain a slight caloric deficit if you're looking to shed fat. If you want to experiment with fasting, do so under controlled circumstances and make sure it fits with your lifestyle and overall goals. But remember, consistency and balance are key, and the idea that you have to skip meals to lose weight is just plain wrong.

Myth #7: "If I Eat That, I'll Get Fat / If I Don't Eat That, I Won't Get Fat"

It's a common misconception that eating certain foods will directly make you gain weight, or conversely, that avoiding certain foods will automatically keep the weight off.

Here's the truth: weight gain or weight loss doesn't happen just from one meal or one snack. It's the overall picture—the balance between what you eat over time and how much you burn through daily activity. That means it's not one food item that's going to make or break your progress.

For example, a slice of cake, an extra burger, or a handful of chips may seem like they'll ruin your progress, but it's not about eating those foods once in a while that leads to weight gain. It's about eating too many calories consistently, over time. A single indulgence won't "make you fat"—just as eating one salad doesn't make you instantly lean.

The Bigger Picture: Calories in vs. Calories out

Let's use the fuel analogy again. Imagine that your body is like a car, and the fuel is the food you eat. If you only put enough fuel in for the trip you're going on (calories consumed equals calories burned), you're fine. But if you keep filling up the tank, even with "healthy" foods, and not burning enough energy, that extra fuel (calories) is stored in your body as fat.

So, whether it's a burger, cake, or a healthy salad, it all comes down to how much you're eating compared to how much energy you're expending. The key is moderation, balance, and overall calorie intake—not demonizing specific foods.

The Real Issue: Focus on Long-Term Habits

Instead of focusing on whether or not a single food will make you fat, it's more important to develop habits that support your long-term goals. Can you manage your calorie intake over time? Can you enjoy that cake occasionally without guilt, while still staying on track with your nutrition?

It's important to remember: it's not about *what* you eat once in a while, but rather *how much* you eat over the course of days, weeks, and months. Focus on consistency, making smart food choices most of the time, and don't sweat the occasional indulgence.

Takeaway:
You can eat everything you like! It's not about avoiding foods, but about moderation and meeting your daily calorie and nutrient needs. Balance is key—if you eat the right portions and stay within your energy requirements, you won't gain weight, regardless of what foods you choose.

Myth #8: "Sweating Like Crazy Means You're Burning Fat"

Ah, the infamous "sweat more, lose more" myth. You've probably heard it before: some people believe that if they're sweating a lot, they're burning fat like crazy. This myth often leads people to extremes, like wearing sauna suits, wrapping themselves in plastic, or even doing intense workouts in the heat. And while it might seem like a good idea—after all, sweat is a sign you're working hard, right?—the truth is far less glamorous.

The Truth:

Sweating is your body's way of cooling itself down. It's not a direct indication that you're burning fat. In fact, the majority of the weight you lose when sweating excessively is **water weight**—not fat. When you exercise intensely or in a hot environment, your body loses fluids in the form of sweat, but once you rehydrate, that weight returns.

This is exactly what happened to your uncle when he told you about his experience. His wife suggested he add a garage sack (or some other form of added heat) while cycling, which made him sweat buckets. He lost weight in the moment, but within an hour of getting back and rehydrating, all that water weight came right back.

Why It's a Myth:

People often mistake water weight loss for fat loss. While sweating may help you drop a few pounds temporarily, it has nothing to do with burning fat. Fat loss, on the other hand, comes from maintaining a caloric deficit over time. You need to burn more calories than you consume, not just sweat excessively.

In reality, focusing on hydration, nutrition, and consistent exercise is far more effective for long-term fat loss than relying on sweat-inducing methods. Your body's natural mechanisms—like sweating—are part of staying healthy, but they're not magical fat-burning tools.

So, ditch the garage sack and instead focus on building sustainable habits: regular workouts (combining cardio and strength training), eating at a caloric deficit, and staying hydrated. You'll lose fat in the long run, not just sweat.

Takeaway:
Sweat doesn't burn fat—calories do. Stay hydrated, focus on your calorie intake, and keep your eye on your long-term goals instead of chasing short-term "sweat" results. Remember, sweating is simply your body's way of cooling down, not an indicator of fat loss.

Myth #9: "You Have to Completely Give Up Your Favorite Foods to Lose Weight"

One of the biggest misconceptions about weight loss is the idea that you have to completely give up the foods you love. Many people believe that if they want to lose weight, they have to say goodbye to pizza, chocolate, burgers, or any of their favorite indulgences. But this couldn't be further from the truth.

Here's the reality: *You don't have to cut out your favorite foods to lose weight.* The key is moderation and balance.

Weight loss is not about complete restriction; it's about creating sustainable habits that fit into your lifestyle. It's more about how you *manage* those favorite foods, rather than entirely eliminating them. You can still enjoy the occasional pizza or piece of chocolate while losing weight, as long as you're mindful of your overall calorie intake.

Moderation is the Secret

Think of it like this: just because you're watching your calorie intake, doesn't mean you have to be miserable or feel deprived. When you *moderate* the amount of your favorite foods, you create a balanced approach that allows you to enjoy life without overindulging. The key is fitting these foods into your daily calorie budget in a way that doesn't prevent you from losing weight.

For example, if you want to enjoy a slice of pizza, you can plan for it by adjusting other parts of your day's meals or exercising a bit more. This way, you're still staying within your overall calorie goal and enjoying the foods you love.

Weighing the Difference

To help understand this concept better, let's use an example: Let's say you're deciding between an apple and a doughnut. We all know an apple is a healthy choice, but you might think that just because a doughnut is more "indulgent," it's out of the question for weight loss. But here's the truth: the calories in the apple and the doughnut are not the same.

An apple has about 90 calories, packed with vitamins and fiber that help keep you full and provide energy. A doughnut, on the other hand, can have around 250–300 calories, loaded with sugar and fat but offering very little in terms of nutrients. So, while the doughnut is higher in calories, it's important to think about *how* those calories fit into your daily intake, rather than just focusing on one item.

In other words, weight loss isn't about banning foods. It's about *balancing* them. You could have the doughnut and work it into your calorie goals by adjusting your other meals, or you could opt for an apple if you're looking for a lighter snack. The difference is how you *manage* the calories, not whether you eat them.

Sustainability is Key

Restricting yourself too much or cutting out entire food groups often leads to feeling deprived, which can make it harder to stick to your diet long-term. When you try to be too rigid, you may end up binging or quitting altogether. In contrast, a more flexible approach allows you to maintain healthy habits without feeling like you're missing out.

The trick is to focus on *long-term sustainability*. Instead of thinking about weight loss as a temporary "diet," think of it as a new way of living—one where you can enjoy your favorite foods in moderation, while still making progress toward your goals.

A Balanced Approach

Eating your favorite foods doesn't mean you have to eat them every day. It's about incorporating them into a healthy, balanced diet, while still prioritizing nutrient-dense foods like fruits, vegetables, whole grains, and lean proteins. It's the overall pattern of what you eat that determines whether you lose weight, not the occasional treat.

So, next time you think about reaching for a chocolate bar or grabbing a burger, remember that losing weight isn't about denying yourself the things you love. It's about finding a balance that works for *you*. By making smart choices, tracking your overall calorie intake, and staying consistent, you can still enjoy your favorite foods and lose weight in a healthy, sustainable way.

Takeaway:
You don't need to give up your favorite foods to lose weight. It's about balance and moderation, not total restriction. Focus on portion control and fitting treats into your overall calorie goals.

Myth #10: "More Exercise = More Weight Loss"

Exercise is crucial for overall health and can contribute to weight loss, but simply increasing your workout time won't automatically lead to fat loss—especially if your diet isn't aligned with your goals.

The reality is that your body is already burning calories just by being alive. This is called your **Basal Metabolic Rate (BMR)**—the number of calories your body needs to maintain basic bodily functions like breathing, circulating blood, and maintaining body temperature, even when you're just sitting still. In fact, BMR typically accounts for around 60-75% of your total daily calorie expenditure! That means that whether you exercise or not, your body is constantly burning calories to keep you functioning.

Exercise does burn calories, of course, but it's often less than people think. You might burn 200-400 calories from a workout session, but if your diet is out of balance, you can easily consume more than that in just one meal.

So, while more exercise can help, weight loss comes down to the balance between calories in (the food you eat) and calories out (the energy your body uses, including exercise). If you're burning 500 calories through exercise but consuming 800 extra calories, you won't lose weight.

The best approach is to combine a balanced diet with exercise. Focus on creating a consistent calorie deficit through diet first, and then add exercise to improve overall fitness and speed up your results.

Takeaway:
More exercise doesn't automatically mean more weight loss. Focus on balancing your diet with exercise to create a consistent calorie deficit. Weight loss is about calories in vs. calories out—simple as that.

Myth #11: "I'm Doing Everything Right, But I'm Still Not Losing Weight"

Tough love time. If you're telling yourself, "I'm eating right, working out, tracking everything, and still not losing weight," here's the truth: don't lie to yourself. You might be able to fool others, but your body doesn't lie.

It's like when you're sitting in the dentist's chair, and they ask if you've been avoiding candy and soda. You might say "yes," but both of you know what's really going on. It's no different with weight loss. You might think you're on point, but those extra bites, occasional indulgences, or half-hearted workouts? They add up.

If you're not seeing results, something's missing. Maybe you're underestimating your calorie intake or overestimating how much you're burning. Be brutally honest with yourself—no excuses. The process works if you work it. So, before you claim that you're doing everything right, take a hard look at what you're really doing.

Exercise: Track Everything Here's your assignment. Download a calorie-tracking app—there are tons of free options on the Play Store or App Store. Track *everything* that goes into your mouth, even those 1-3 almonds you grab on the way to the couch. Every sip, every bite—log it. You'll be surprised how quickly those "little" things add up. This exercise will help you get a crystal-clear picture of your actual intake and show you where adjustments can be made.

Don't lie to yourself. If you're serious about results, get serious about owning the process.

Takeaway:
No excuses. Stop lying to yourself—track everything, be brutally honest, and own the process. Results come when you do the work, no shortcuts.

Myth #12: "I Need to Do a Juice Cleanse or Detox to Lose Weight"

Let's get one thing straight: juice cleanses, detox teas, and all those "quick fix" solutions are pure BS. These fads make it sound like your body is full of toxins and that the only way to get rid of them is to starve yourself on a liquid diet for a week. But guess what? Your body already has a perfectly good detox system in place—it's called your liver and kidneys. They're working 24/7 to keep you clean and healthy.

Juice cleanses may help you drop a few pounds, but it's not fat you're losing—it's **water weight** and **muscle mass**, and often the few nutrients you were getting. And once you start eating solid food again, those pounds come right back. On top of that, these cleanses can leave you feeling weak, dizzy, and completely drained because you're depriving your body of the protein, fats, and carbs it actually needs to function.

Weight loss isn't about flushing out so-called toxins with a $50 cleanse—it's about eating real, balanced meals and sticking to a sustainable calorie deficit. Detoxing? That's just marketing hype designed to drain your wallet, not your body fat.

Save yourself the headache (literally) and ditch the juice cleanses. Focus on a balanced diet that supports your body's natural detox system and gives you the fuel you need to power through your day.

Takeaway: Juices and detoxes won't give you long-term results. Stick to real food, real nutrition, and real results.

Closing Thoughts: Debunking the Lies

At the end of the day, weight loss isn't a magic trick or a quick fix—it's a process that requires real commitment, self-awareness, and consistency. The myths we've debunked here are just a few of the many misleading ideas that make their way into the world of fitness and weight loss. Remember, the road to real, lasting results is built on facts, not fantasy.

So, stop chasing the next quick fix or trying to cut corners. Instead, focus on what works—calorie balance, proper nutrition, consistent exercise, and mental toughness. Every one of those so-called "hacks" or "secret formulas" you've heard about? They're distractions from the real goal.

The truth is, there's no easy way to achieve sustainable weight loss. There's no shortcut, and there's no special food or exercise routine that will get you there faster. The truth is, you need to stay consistent, trust the process, and get serious about your health. The best way to lose weight, feel strong, and build lasting habits is by taking an honest, straightforward approach.

Now that you've separated the facts from the fiction, it's time to get serious and make your progress real. Let's move forward.

The Science Behind Fat Loss

Introduction to Fat Loss

Key Concept: Fat Loss is All About Calorie Balance

When it comes to losing fat, there's no magic formula. It all comes down to **calorie balance**—the relationship between the calories you take in and the calories you burn. Simply put, fat loss is achieved when you burn **more calories than you consume**.

Think of your body like a car engine. **Fuel** is the food and drink you consume, while your body's energy needs to keep running are the calories burned. Just like a car needs the right amount of fuel to run efficiently, your body needs the right balance of calories to maintain, gain, or lose weight.

If you put in too much fuel (calories) for the engine (your body), it'll start to overflow, just like gaining weight. If you don't put in enough fuel, the engine won't run properly, and your body will slow down. The right balance is essential.

We touched on this earlier in the book when we talked about how **your body burns calories** and uses energy, so keep this fuel analogy in mind as we go deeper into the science of fat loss.

Energy Balance: Calories In vs. Calories Out

At the core of fat loss is the concept of **energy balance**. Every day, your body is either in a state of calorie **surplus** (eating more than you burn) or calorie **deficit** (burning more than you eat). Here's the basic equation:

- **Calories In**: The energy (fuel) you get from food and drinks.

- **Calories Out**: The energy your body burns through bodily functions, exercise, and physical activity.

To lose fat, you need to be in a **calorie deficit**—meaning you're burning more calories than you're taking in. This is the key to fat loss, and it's as simple as that.

Basal Metabolic Rate (BMR): The Engine Behind Fat Loss

Your body is constantly using energy, even when you're at rest. This energy expenditure is called **Basal Metabolic Rate (BMR)**. It accounts for the largest portion of your daily calorie burn—typically around 60-75% of your total energy expenditure.

Think of BMR as the idle power of your body's engine. It's the energy your body needs to maintain basic life-sustaining functions, such as:

- Breathing
- Circulating blood
- Maintaining body temperature
- Digesting food
- Other vital processes like cellular repair and brain function

In short, **BMR** is the minimum number of calories your body requires to function at rest.

Total Daily Energy Expenditure (TDEE): Your True Maintenance Level

While BMR is important, it's only part of the equation. Your body also burns calories from **exercise**, physical activity, and even simple activities like walking or standing (which is known as **NEAT**: Non-Exercise Activity Thermogenesis).

When you add up BMR and all these activities, you get your **Total Daily Energy Expenditure (TDEE)**. TDEE represents the total number of calories your body needs to maintain its current weight, considering all the physical activity you engage in.

Here's a quick overview:

- **TDEE = BMR + calories burned from physical activity (exercise, walking, fidgeting, etc.)**

How to Create a Calorie Deficit

To lose fat, you need to **create a calorie deficit**. That means consuming fewer calories than your TDEE. For example, if your TDEE is 2,500 calories, and you eat 2,000 calories a day, you've created a **500-calorie deficit**.

It's simple:

- **500 calories per day x 7 days = 3,500 calories per week.**
- Since **3,500 calories equals about 1 pound of fat**, a 500-calorie daily deficit will lead to the loss of approximately **1 pound of fat per week**.

The Bottom Line

Fat loss boils down to understanding and managing your calorie balance. **Burn more calories than you consume, and you'll lose fat.** Just like a car engine burns fuel to run, your body burns calories for energy. The challenge is to ensure you're giving it the right amount of fuel and using it efficiently.

In the next section, we'll dive deeper into the science behind how calories are burned, and how you can apply these principles to maximize fat loss while maintaining your health.

How Fat Loss Works: Mechanisms of Fat Loss

Fat loss isn't just a simple equation of calories in versus calories out. While calorie balance is crucial, the process of fat loss involves complex mechanisms within your body. From hormones to fat mobilization and energy utilization, understanding how fat is burned will help you optimize your fat loss journey.

The Role of Hormones in Fat Loss

Hormones are the chemical messengers that regulate your body's functions, including fat storage and appetite. The following hormones play a critical role in fat loss:

- **Insulin**: After eating, your body releases insulin to help store excess energy. While insulin is essential for nutrient storage, it also promotes fat storage by signaling fat cells to retain energy. Consuming high-carb or sugary meals frequently can spike insulin and promote fat gain. To lose fat, controlling insulin levels through balanced carb intake is key.

- **Leptin**: Known as the "satiety hormone," leptin signals to your brain that you're full and have enough energy. Higher leptin levels reduce hunger, while lower leptin levels increase it. During a calorie deficit (when losing fat), leptin levels drop, causing an increase in hunger. Combat this by eating nutrient-dense, satisfying foods to stay full and manage hunger better.

- **Cortisol**: Cortisol, the stress hormone, can hinder fat loss by promoting fat storage, especially in the abdominal area. Chronic stress can elevate cortisol levels, making fat loss more challenging. Managing stress through techniques like relaxation and quality sleep helps support a healthy metabolism.

Fat Mobilization: Breaking Down Fat for Energy

Your body doesn't just magically burn fat when you create a calorie deficit. The process is more involved and requires your body to go through **lipolysis**, where stored fat is broken down into usable energy:

- **Lipolysis**: When you're in a calorie deficit, your body releases fat from fat cells. The fat is broken down into **free fatty acids** and **glycerol**, which are then transported through your bloodstream to be used as energy.

- **Fatty Acid Oxidation**: These free fatty acids are carried to muscles and other tissues where they are burned for fuel. This process, known as **fatty acid oxidation**, takes place primarily during lower-intensity activities, like walking or steady-state cardio. It helps fuel your body, especially when in a calorie deficit.

Energy Use: How Fat Powers Your Body

Your body is constantly using energy for basic functions and physical activity. Fat plays a crucial role in this energy production, particularly when you're in a calorie deficit:

- **Resting Energy Expenditure**: Even when you're resting, your body uses energy to maintain vital functions such as breathing, circulating blood, and regulating body temperature. This means you're burning calories even when not exercising.

- **Exercise**: Physical activity increases energy expenditure. Exercise, especially a combination of **strength training** and **cardio**, helps increase the number of calories burned each day. During exercise, fat becomes one of the main sources of fuel, particularly during **low to moderate-intensity** activities.

Types of Fat: Subcutaneous vs. Visceral Fat

Not all fat is created equal. There are two key types of fat in your body, each playing a different role:

- **Subcutaneous Fat**: This is the fat you can pinch under your skin. It's the most common type of fat and is often the first to be burned during weight loss. Subcutaneous fat is generally less harmful than visceral fat.

- **Visceral Fat**: This type of fat is stored deeper in your body, around your organs. It is associated with serious health risks like heart disease and diabetes. However, it's also the first fat to be mobilized and burned when you lose weight. As you shed pounds, visceral fat tends to decrease early in the process.

The Takeaway: Fat Loss Is Complex, But Achievable

Fat loss is a complex process, but at its core, it's about balancing energy. Hormones, fat mobilization, and energy use all work together to help your body burn fat. By understanding these mechanisms, you'll be better equipped to optimize your fat loss approach, ensuring you're not just losing weight, but effectively burning fat and improving your body composition.

In the next section, we'll explore why "spot reduction" is a myth and why you can't lose fat from specific areas of your body by targeting them with exercises. Fat loss happens uniformly across your body, not in one targeted area.

Fat Burning vs. Fat Loss

Fat burning and fat loss are often used interchangeably, but they're not exactly the same thing. Understanding the difference is key to optimizing your fat loss approach and avoiding confusion around trendy diets or fitness fads.

Fat Burning vs. Fat Loss: What's the Difference?

When your body burns fat, it's simply using fat as a source of energy. This happens constantly throughout the day, whether you're exercising or just going about your daily activities. But burning fat doesn't automatically mean you're losing fat from your body—fat loss is a much more specific process.

Fat loss occurs when your body is in a **calorie deficit**, meaning you burn more calories than you consume, leading to a reduction in stored fat over time. So, while fat burning is part of the process, fat loss is what you're after when it comes to losing weight.

Now, let's dive into the role of **fat as fuel**, especially with diets like keto and low-carb diets, and how they influence the body's ability to burn fat.

Fat as Fuel: How Low-Carb and Keto Diets Promote Fat Burning

While your body normally relies on carbohydrates for quick energy, it can shift into **fat-burning mode** if you restrict carbs sufficiently. This is where diets like **ketogenic (keto)** and **low-carb** come into play. These diets change how your body sources its energy, forcing it to use fat as its primary fuel instead of carbs.

1. **Keto Diet**: By drastically reducing carbs (usually to less than 50 grams a day), the body enters **ketosis**—a state where the body burns fat for fuel rather than glucose (from carbohydrates). As your body begins to break down fat, it produces **ketones**, which provide energy for your brain and muscles.
    This process results in **fat burning** but can lead to **fat loss** if you're still in a calorie deficit. The body burns fat for energy, but if you're eating too many calories, you won't lose the fat stored in your body.

2. **Low-Carb Diet**: While not as extreme as keto, a low-carb diet still reduces your body's reliance on carbs for energy. With fewer carbs, your body starts burning fat at a higher rate for fuel, but it's still important to maintain a caloric deficit for fat loss to occur.

So while **fat burning** can happen with these diets, **fat loss** only occurs if you're consuming fewer calories than you burn over time. These diets help with fat burning by switching your energy source, but they don't automatically lead to fat loss without a proper calorie deficit.

The Role of Calories: Fuel and Energy Management

As mentioned earlier, your body is like an engine, and just like a car, it needs the right type and amount of fuel. Fat can certainly be a key fuel source, especially on low-carb and ketogenic diets. But whether you're using fat or carbohydrates for energy, the most important thing is **calorie balance**.

*   **Calories In**: The food you eat provides energy.
*   **Calories Out**: Your body burns energy through metabolism, exercise, and daily activities.

To **lose fat**, you need to create a calorie deficit. Whether you're burning fat through exercise, on a ketogenic diet, or through everyday activities, it's the deficit that determines fat loss. Fat burning is a natural process, but fat loss is a result of consistently using more energy than you consume.

Key Takeaway: Fat Burning vs. Fat Loss

Fat burning and fat loss are different but interconnected processes. Fat burning happens as your body breaks down fat to use as fuel, and this happens whether you're on a high-carb or low-carb diet. But fat loss—the reduction in stored body fat—happens when you burn more calories than you consume, whether that's by eating less, moving more, or both.

So, while diets like keto and low-carb diets can promote fat burning by switching your body's fuel source to fat, **the key to fat loss remains the same**: creating a consistent calorie deficit. Fat burning might be happening, but fat loss won't occur unless you're managing your calorie intake properly.

In the latter part of the book, we'll dive deeper into specific diets like keto and low-carb and how they can fit into a fat loss strategy. We'll explore the pros and cons of these approaches and how they align with the overall principles of fat loss we're covering.

The Role of Muscle in Fat Loss

When it comes to fat loss, many people focus almost exclusively on **calories burned** and the **calorie deficit**. While that's certainly a critical part of the equation, there's another crucial factor that can significantly impact how effectively and efficiently you burn fat: **muscle mass**.

Muscle Mass: Your Fat-Burning Furnace

Muscle is more than just something that makes you look toned and strong. In fact, muscle plays a key role in fat loss because it **burns more calories at rest** than fat tissue. The more muscle you have, the higher your **resting metabolic rate (RMR)**—meaning, your body burns more calories even when you're not exercising.

Here's why:

- **Muscle burns more energy**: Even when you're not active, muscle tissue requires more energy to maintain than fat tissue. This means that the more muscle you have, the more calories your body will burn throughout the day, just to maintain its current state.

- **Boosting your metabolism**: Building muscle through strength training not only increases your daily energy expenditure, but it also creates an afterburn effect known as **Excess Post-Exercise Oxygen Consumption (EPOC)**. This means your body continues to burn calories after a workout, as it works to recover and repair muscles.

How Strength Training Affects Fat Loss

Many people mistakenly believe that cardio is the only way to burn fat, but strength training is equally, if not more, important when it comes to sustainable fat loss. Here's how:

1. **Increases muscle mass**: Strength training helps you build lean muscle, and as mentioned above, more muscle means a higher metabolic rate. This means that even when you're not working out, you're still burning more calories.

2. **Boosts calorie burn during workouts**: Lifting weights burns calories during your workout, but more importantly, it increases your post-workout calorie burn (EPOC). Strength training also raises your heart rate, helping you burn more calories overall compared to lower-intensity cardio sessions.

3. **Preserves muscle while in a deficit**: When you're in a calorie deficit (eating fewer calories than your body needs to maintain weight), there's a risk of losing muscle along with fat. Strength training helps preserve muscle mass while you're losing fat, ensuring that the majority of weight you lose is fat, not muscle. Without strength training, your body is more likely to break down muscle tissue for energy.

4. **Improves body composition**: While you may see the scale go down during fat loss, it doesn't always reflect the improvement in **body composition** (the ratio of muscle to fat). Strength training helps you maintain or even increase muscle mass, resulting in a leaner, more toned physique, even if your weight doesn't drop drastically. This is why the scale isn't the only indicator of progress.

Fat Loss Isn't Just About Losing Weight

Remember, fat loss is not just about seeing a lower number on the scale. It's about changing **your body composition**—reducing fat while maintaining or increasing muscle. This is why you may lose fat and still see little or no change in the scale. Your body is simply replacing fat with muscle, which is denser and more compact.

A **toned** physique comes from a combination of fat loss and muscle development. **Muscle helps you burn fat**, and the more muscle you build, the easier it is to maintain a healthy body composition, even after you've reached your fat loss goals.

The Role of Resistance Training in Fat Loss

Resistance training, often referred to as strength training, is one of the most effective ways to stimulate muscle growth and promote fat loss. It includes activities like:

- Weight lifting
- Bodyweight exercises (push-ups, squats)
- Resistance bands
- Gym machines

In addition to increasing muscle mass, resistance training also:

- Improves **bone density** (important for overall health as you age)
- Enhances **joint mobility** and stability
- Increases **functional strength**, making everyday tasks easier

Incorporating resistance training into your workout routine is essential for maximizing fat loss and achieving a lean, toned body. It's not just about burning calories during the workout—it's about the long-term impact that increased muscle mass has on your metabolism and fat-burning potential.

Muscle and Fat Loss: The Bigger Picture

To truly understand the relationship between muscle and fat loss, think of your body like a furnace. **Muscle is the fuel that keeps the fire going**, and the more muscle you have, the hotter that furnace burns. This means you're burning more calories 24/7, even when you're not working out, sleeping, or eating.

- **More muscle, more calorie burn**: Even at rest, muscle burns more calories than fat, making it a powerful asset in your fat loss journey.
- **Muscle helps you maintain fat loss**: When you build muscle, you're creating a more metabolically active body, which helps prevent the rebound weight gain that can happen after you've lost fat.

The more muscle you have, the more fat your body will burn both during exercise and while you go about your daily life.

The Takeaway

Muscle is an essential factor in fat loss, and building muscle should be a priority for anyone serious about losing fat. Strength training not only **burns calories during exercise** but also **increases your metabolism** in the long run, helping you burn more calories at rest.

If you focus on building muscle through consistent resistance training while managing your calorie intake, you'll create an environment that promotes **long-term fat loss**, not just temporary weight loss. Combining strength training with a balanced approach to diet and cardio is the key to achieving lasting results, a toned physique, and a higher metabolism.

Conclusion: Understanding Fat Loss Is Key to Success

Fat loss can seem like a daunting and complex process, but at its core, it's really about understanding a few key principles: **calorie balance, energy expenditure**, and the role of **muscle**. By grasping these fundamental concepts, you'll be better equipped to approach fat loss in a sustainable and effective way, without falling for myths or quick-fix solutions.

Here's a quick recap of the key points we've covered:

- **Calorie Balance**: Fat loss comes down to the simple equation of **calories in versus calories out**. To lose fat, you need to be in a calorie deficit—burning more calories than you consume. This means you must focus on both your diet and your activity level to create the right conditions for fat loss.

- **Metabolism**: Your body burns calories to maintain basic functions (BMR) and to power your daily activities (TDEE). The more muscle you have, the more calories you burn at rest, which is why strength training is an essential part of the fat loss equation.

- **Hormones**: Your body's hormonal regulation plays a huge role in fat storage and fat burning. Hormones like insulin, leptin, and cortisol can either help or hinder your fat loss journey, depending on how well you manage your diet, stress, and overall health.

- **Fat Mobilization**: Fat loss isn't just about burning calories—it's also about mobilizing stored fat to be used as energy. Through processes like lipolysis and fatty acid oxidation, your body taps into fat stores and converts them into usable energy.

- **The Role of Muscle**: Muscle is your body's natural fat-burning furnace. The more muscle you build, the higher your metabolism, and the more calories you burn even when you're at rest. Strength training should be a cornerstone of your fat loss plan because it helps preserve muscle, enhances your metabolism, and improves body composition.

The Role of Mindset

Weight Loss Starts in Your Mind

Many people fail at weight loss because they approach it with the wrong mindset. They see it as a temporary fix—a 30-day challenge or a 12-week program—that they can "complete" and then move on. But real weight loss, the kind that lasts, starts with the mind. It's about committing to a lifestyle change, not a short-term solution.

When I set out to write this book, I didn't just aim to teach you how to lose fat and then call it a day. My goal is bigger than that. I want to show you that **for this to work**, you have to **change your life for the better**. You're not just dropping pounds—you're building a stronger mindset, improving your discipline, and creating habits that will serve you in all areas of life.

The truth is, weight loss isn't a quick project. It's something that takes time, patience, and most importantly, a shift in how you think. When you treat weight loss like a temporary challenge, you set yourself up to fail the moment that challenge ends. When you view it as a long-term commitment, you start to focus on building habits that you can maintain for life.

I want to teach you the **discipline** that will not only help you shed fat but also give you the tools to maintain a healthy, balanced lifestyle in the long run.

Mindset Shift: Long-Term Commitment, Not a Quick Fix

This is the first critical shift in mindset: **Weight loss is a marathon, not a sprint.**

You have to think of it as a **lifestyle shift**. Instead of saying, "I want to lose 5kg in 3 weeks," start thinking, "I want to build a lifestyle where I can maintain a healthy weight year-round." This shift in thinking makes all the difference. It changes the way you approach challenges and setbacks. Instead of seeing a single bad day or a cheat meal as a failure, you begin to see the bigger picture and trust the process.

Now, don't get me wrong. **Saying 'I want to lose 5kg in 3 weeks' is not bad**. In fact, **setting goals** is one of the most important factors in achieving success. However, what truly separates those who succeed from those who don't is the ability to **follow through** with those goals. The discipline to stay committed, even when things get tough, is what will carry you across the finish line—not just for those 3 weeks, but for a lifetime.

The Power of Consistency

One of the biggest reasons people fail in weight loss is that they aim for **perfection** instead of **consistency**.

The truth is, no one is perfect. Not even the fittest people you see on social media. But those who succeed in fitness and weight loss are the ones who stay consistent. They might slip up, miss workouts, or have cheat meals, but they always get back on track. **Consistency over time beats perfection every single day**.

You don't have to be perfect. You just have to **keep going**. Even if you mess up, even if you don't feel like it some days—what matters is showing up day in and day out.

Like we mentioned earlier, too many people set big, short-term goals: "I want to lose 4kg in a week." Why doesn't anyone plan for the long-term? Why not set a goal like, "I want to see how much I can lose in 1 year"? That kind of goal is exciting, mysterious, and alluring. It shifts the focus from quick fixes to **discovering your full potential** over time. It's not just about weight loss, but about who you become in the process.

Visualization and Positive Thinking

Visualization is a powerful tool in weight loss. When you visualize yourself achieving your goals, you're more likely to stay motivated and work toward them. Take a moment to picture yourself with the body you want or with the health and energy you're striving for. **Feel it.** Hold onto that feeling when times get tough.

Positive thinking plays a role, too. Instead of focusing on how far you have to go, focus on the **positive progress** you're making. Every small step matters, and it's important to celebrate those small wins. Whether it's a drop in weight, an improvement in strength, or just feeling more energetic—those are all victories.

Adopt the mindset: **I can, I want, I will.** You've already made it this far into the book! Ask yourself: are you done with the excuses? **START NOW!** You don't need to wait for the perfect time, or for everything to fall into place—just take action today. Every step forward, no matter how small, brings you closer to your goal.

Visualize, think positive, and take action. It's that simple.

Handling Setbacks

Setbacks are part of the journey. They are **inevitable**, and anyone who tells you otherwise isn't being honest. The key difference between people who succeed and those who don't is their ability to handle setbacks.

Instead of letting one bad day ruin your entire plan, learn to **get back on track quickly**. One bad meal doesn't mean you've ruined your diet, and one missed workout doesn't erase your progress. The **only failure** is quitting. Keep that in mind whenever you feel discouraged.

That's life! Sometimes things are out of your control—**business meetings, kids' soccer practice,** or other obligations might throw you off. But skipping one workout doesn't undo your efforts. However, **skipping 5 workouts, drowning yourself in beer and burgers for days in a row—now you're just fucking around again.** That's the difference between an occasional slip and falling off the wagon completely.

Remember, setbacks don't define you. **How you respond to them does.** Don't let a small stumble derail your progress—**get back on track** and keep moving forward.

Conclusion: Mindset is Everything

In weight loss, **your mind is your most powerful tool**. It's what will carry you through the tough days, help you push past setbacks, and keep you focused on your long-term goals.

Without the right mindset, no amount of diets or workouts will work. But with it, you can achieve lasting success.

Do you know how many times people have **looked at me weird** because I said no to cake or sweets? I don't need them. The crazy part is how **unimportant these types of food** become when you start taking things seriously. I haven't had cake for six months, and guess what? There's **nothing** that pushes me to have some.

Remember, I'm not teaching you to stop eating cake or any specific food. I'm telling you how **banal these foods become** when you take them off the pedestal you've put them on. They lose their power over you when they're no longer treated like a reward or indulgence. Once you remove the emotional attachment, they're just another food you can take or leave.

When you shift your mindset, the things that once felt like a sacrifice—skipping dessert or avoiding junk food—become effortless. **Discipline** starts to feel like freedom. It's not about deprivation; it's about building habits that align with your goals and, ultimately, your happiness.

Mindset is everything. Nail this, and the rest will follow.

Action Steps: Putting the Truth into Practice

Now that we've covered the **truth about weight loss** and the mindset it requires, it's time to get down to action. The truth is, all the knowledge in the world is useless without implementation. This chapter is about **putting the truth into practice**. Here are some simple, no-nonsense steps to get you started with weight loss today—**the real, sustainable way**.

Simple First Steps

1. Calculate Your Maintenance Calories and Establish a Calorie Deficit

Before you can lose weight, you need to understand how much energy (calories) your body requires to maintain its current weight. This is called your **maintenance calories**. Once you know this, the next step is to establish a **calorie deficit**—meaning you need to consume fewer calories than you burn. Here's how to do it:

- **Step 1:** Use an online calculator to determine your daily calorie needs based on your age, weight, height, and activity level.
- **Step 2:** Aim for a small **calorie deficit** of 300-500 calories per day. This will lead to a steady weight loss of around 0.5-1kg per week, which is a healthy and sustainable rate.

Tip: Don't go overboard with the deficit. A large calorie cut can lead to energy loss, poor performance in the gym, and an increased likelihood of binge eating. **Moderation is key.**

2. Incorporate Whole Foods Into Your Meals

One of the simplest and most effective changes you can make is to start eating **whole foods**— foods that are minimally processed and closest to their natural state. Think of foods like:

- **Lean proteins:** Chicken, turkey, fish, eggs, tofu, etc.
- **Fruits and vegetables:** Fresh produce, not sugary snacks.
- **Healthy fats:** Avocados, nuts, seeds, olive oil, etc.

Why? Whole foods are nutrient-dense and help you feel full longer. They provide the vitamins and minerals your body needs for optimal performance, recovery, and fat loss. Plus, they're much less likely to cause overeating compared to processed foods that are high in added sugars and unhealthy fats.

3. Begin a Basic Strength Training Routine (2-3 Times Per Week)

Strength training isn't a requirement for weight loss, but it helps **a lot**. If you want to lose weight, you don't **have** to lift weights or hit the gym. But, if you do include strength training in your routine, it can make a **big difference** in how your body looks and how fast you lose fat.

Here's why it helps:

- **It boosts metabolism**: Building muscle increases your resting metabolic rate (RMR), meaning you burn more calories even when you're not working out.
- **It preserves muscle mass**: When you're in a calorie deficit, strength training ensures that the weight you lose comes from fat, not muscle.

How to get started:

If you decide to include it, you don't need to get fancy with expensive gym equipment:

- Choose basic, compound movements like squats, push-ups, lunges, and rows. These work multiple muscle groups and are easy to do at home.
- Start with 2-3 full-body workouts per week. You don't need to lift heavy or do complex exercises to see results.
- Focus on getting stronger over time, either by increasing the weight or the number of reps.

Tip: Strength training is great for building muscle and improving how you feel in the long run, but **it's not mandatory**. If you're not into it, no worries—weight loss can still happen without lifting a single weight. However, if you do decide to give it a shot, consistency with strength training can really **transform your body composition** over time.

While the scale might not move dramatically at first, remember: muscle is more **dense** than fat. As you build muscle, the scale may even go up a bit. But don't let that discourage you! Focus on progress over numbers—how you feel, your strength, energy, and how your clothes fit matter way more than the scale.

4. Add in 20-30 Minutes of Moderate Cardio (3-4 Times Per Week)

Cardio can be an important part of the equation, but it's not the only tool for fat loss. In fact, strength training should be your primary focus. However, **moderate cardio** can still help you burn extra calories and improve overall fitness.

- **Low-impact options:** Walking, cycling, swimming, or using an elliptical machine.
- **Higher-intensity options:** Jogging, running, rowing, or high-intensity interval training (HIIT).

Tip: Cardio should feel like an addition, not a requirement. If you enjoy it, do it! But if you don't, don't force it. You can still lose fat with just strength training and a good diet. **Cardio is optional.**

5. Emphasize Consistency

Consistency is where most people fail. They go all-in, push hard, but when they miss a workout or overeat, they throw in the towel and quit entirely. Instead of aiming for perfection, focus on **being consistent**.

You don't need to be perfect. The truth is, you're going to have off days. You might miss a workout, or have a meal that isn't exactly aligned with your plan. That's okay. What matters is that you **keep going**.

Even when you don't feel like working out or you have a meal that doesn't fit your ideal plan, show up. Every time you show up, even when it's tough, you're building resilience and discipline. It's those small, consistent actions that matter most in the long run.

Set a goal to be consistent for at least 3-4 weeks before evaluating your progress. This will give your body time to adjust, allow your new habits to solidify, and help shift your mindset. Instead of looking for quick results, give yourself the time to make real, sustainable changes.

And when it comes to weighing yourself, **don't sweat the small fluctuations.** Weigh yourself at the end of the week and see where you're at. If your weight has gone down, that's a win. If it's gone up, that's still a win. It means your body is adjusting, and you're making progress, even if the scale doesn't reflect it right away.

Don't let weight fluctuations derail you. The scale is just one piece of the puzzle. Your real success is in the habits you're building and the consistent efforts you're making. Keep moving forward, even when you don't see drastic changes right away.

Stick with it. Consistency always pays off in the end.

PS: If you follow everything I've mentioned so far, I **guarantee** you will lose weight. I'm so confident in this that I'd bet my car, my house, and everything else on it! The principles I've laid out are proven, straightforward, and real. Stick to them, stay consistent, and you'll see the results—no excuses, no shortcuts.

6. Focus on Small Wins

It's easy to get frustrated when you don't see immediate results, but weight loss is not about quick fixes. It's about **small wins over time**. The process may not always be fast, but every little step counts. These small, consistent efforts lead to real, lasting change.

Celebrate every victory, no matter how small. Whether it's:

- Eating a balanced meal.
- Completing your workout for the day.

- Getting enough sleep.
- Losing a fraction of a kilogram on the scale.

Every small win counts. These are all steps in the right direction. The key is to **not obsess over the scale** or try to "rush" the process. Don't get discouraged by the slow pace. **Trust the process**, and celebrate every success along the way.

And here's a simple, yet powerful tip: **Just leave the cake alone. Let it rot.** You don't need it right now. You can eat it tomorrow—heck, you can let it rot and eat it next week. In the meantime, focus on your goals, on how far you've come, and on the victories that matter more than that momentary craving. **You are in control.**

It's about teaching yourself the discipline to **stay the course**, even when it feels tempting to give in. This is how you build a foundation for long-term success, not by succumbing to every craving, but by showing yourself that you have the power to say no when it matters. **Let the cake wait.**

To Sum It Up:

- **Step 1:** Calculate your maintenance calories and create a modest calorie deficit.
- **Step 2:** Incorporate more whole foods—lean proteins, fruits, vegetables, and healthy fats.
- **Step 3:** Start strength training 2-3 times a week.
- **Step 4:** Add 20-30 minutes of moderate cardio (if you enjoy it).
- **Step 5:** Be consistent for at least 3-4 weeks before reassessing.
- **Step 6:** Focus on small wins and don't let the scale be your only measure of success.

This is where **real results** happen. It's about getting started and sticking with it, even when things get tough. You don't need to have it all figured out right now, just take the first step and trust the process. **The consistency will pay off.**

As we move forward in this book, I'll cover workout plans, variations, and cardio in greater detail. If you're curious about those, just refer to the index to find the relevant sections. Remember, the journey of weight loss is ongoing, and each step you take brings you closer to your goals!

Conclusion: The Real Work Begins Now

Wrap-Up:

You've made it this far, and that's a huge win. But let's be honest: this is just the beginning. Now, it's time to put the truth into action.

The most important things you need to keep in mind are **mindset** and **consistency**. Without the right mindset, no amount of diet plans, workout routines, or supplements will help you get results. Your mind is the foundation, and when you treat weight loss as a lifestyle change rather than a quick fix, you're setting yourself up for lasting success.

But here's the truth: **results don't happen overnight.** It takes time, patience, and persistence. The hardest part of the process isn't getting started—it's sticking with it, even when things don't go exactly as planned. You might have bad days, slip-ups, and moments where progress feels slow. But that's all part of the journey. What matters is your commitment to the long haul.

Remember, the real work is making fitness and healthy living a permanent part of your life. It's about creating habits that will support your goals day after day, week after week, and month after month. The key to lasting weight loss isn't in a 30-day challenge or a quick fad diet—it's in the small, consistent actions you take over time.

Don't get distracted by the scale or short-term results. Focus on creating **sustainable habits**— the things you can do every day, without feeling like you're sacrificing or forcing yourself to do something that isn't realistic for you. Small victories—like choosing a balanced meal, getting enough sleep, or sticking to your workout plan for the week—will add up over time, and that's when the magic happens.

I want you to **commit to the long haul**. This isn't a sprint, and it's not about quick fixes. It's about developing the discipline and mindset that will help you stay on track, no matter what life throws at you.

So, now that you know the truth about weight loss, it's time to put it into practice. You've got the tools, the knowledge, and the plan. The real challenge? Staying consistent and being patient. But I know you can do it. **Trust the process.**

Be patient. Be consistent. And above all, **keep showing up**—because that's where the real transformation happens.

Chapter 2: The No BS Diet: What to Eat for Weight Loss

In this chapter, we're not going to get bogged down in rigid meal plans or complicated rules. Instead, I'm going to show you how to make eating for weight loss simple and effective. The No BS Diet is about real-life strategies you can apply, without all the unnecessary hype or restrictions.

The Truth About Nutrition

There's no secret diet or magic food that will shed the pounds for you. The truth is simple: weight loss comes down to eating fewer calories than you burn while still nourishing your body with the right balance of macronutrients (protein, carbs, fats) and micronutrients (vitamins and minerals).

The No BS approach to nutrition is focused on simplicity, flexibility, and long-term sustainability. Here's how to make it work for you.

1. Food Categories: Building Blocks of a Weight loss Diet

Instead of giving you a strict meal plan, let's focus on food categories that you can incorporate into your diet. Aim to eat foods that are nutrient-dense and fuel your body for performance and fat loss.

Proteins

Protein is essential for fat loss and muscle preservation, especially when you're in a calorie deficit. It helps keep you feeling full and supports muscle repair after workouts. Here are some examples of high-quality protein sources:

- **Lean meats** (chicken, turkey)
- **Fish and seafood** (salmon, tuna)
- **Eggs and egg whites**
- **Plant-based proteins** (tofu, tempeh, lentils)
- **Greek yogurt or cottage cheese**

Carbohydrates

Carbs are the body's main energy source, so you need them, but choose **complex carbs** that keep you fuller longer and don't spike your blood sugar. Opt for whole-food sources that provide fiber and nutrients. Here are good options:

- **Vegetables** (especially leafy greens)
- **Whole grains** (brown rice, quinoa, oats)
- **Fruits** (berries, apples, oranges)
- **Sweet potatoes and legumes**

Fats

Healthy fats are crucial for hormone function and energy. While fats are more calorie-dense, they are necessary for overall health, so don't shy away from them entirely. Just be mindful of portions. Here are examples of healthy fats:

- **Avocado**
- **Olive oil or coconut oil**
- **Nuts and seeds**
- **Fatty fish** (salmon, sardines)

These categories give you the freedom to build balanced meals without overcomplicating things. You don't need to count every calorie or weigh your food—just focus on eating from these nutrient-dense categories, and you'll be on the right path for sustainable fat loss.

2. How to Build Your Own Meals (No Bullshit)

We don't need to complicate things with detailed meal plans. Here's how you can easily build your meals for fat loss, muscle building, or simply maintaining a balanced diet.

Focus on Balance

Each meal should include a good source of **protein, complex carbs,** and **healthy fats.** This balance will keep you full, energized, and help you stay on track with your goals. Here's a breakdown of what to focus on:

Use the Plate Method:

- **Option 1:**
  Half your plate should be **veggies**, a quarter should be **protein**, and the last quarter should be **carbs**. This method helps you keep calories lower while still making sure you're getting the nutrients you need to feel full and satisfied. Focus on nutrient-dense, low-calorie foods like leafy greens, non-starchy vegetables, and whole grains.

    - **Veggies**: Leafy greens (spinach, kale, lettuce), broccoli, cauliflower, peppers, cucumbers, etc.
    - **Protein**: Lean meats (chicken, turkey), fish, eggs, Greek yogurt, tofu, or legumes like lentils.
    - **Carbs**: Whole grains (brown rice, quinoa, oats), sweet potatoes, or beans and legumes.

- **Option 2: Higher Protein Intake**
  Aim for **half your plate** to be **protein, a quarter to veggies**, and **a quarter to carbs**. This method is ideal if you want to focus on muscle repair and higher protein intake to support recovery and growth. You can still include healthy fats, but make sure they're in moderation.

    - **Protein**: More protein-rich foods like chicken breast, lean beef, fish, eggs, protein powders, Greek yogurt, or cottage cheese. If you're plant-based, tofu, tempeh, lentils, and beans work great.
    - **Veggies**: Non-starchy vegetables such as spinach, zucchini, mushrooms, and green beans are great options.
    - **Carbs**: Carbs like quinoa, brown rice, whole wheat bread, and oats will provide energy for your workouts and recovery.

Portion Control: Don't Overcomplicate It

No need to obsess over exact calorie counts or macros. The key is learning how much to eat to fuel your body without going overboard. When in doubt, follow the plate method as a simple guideline. Eat until you're satisfied, but not overly full.

What Should You Eat?

Here's the No BS truth: Eating for fat loss doesn't have to be complicated, and it certainly doesn't mean giving up the foods you enjoy. But we're also going to remove these foods from their pedestal. There's nothing "special" about a Snickers, muffin, or a Coke. They're just calories, like everything else.

Nutrient-Dense Foods: Your Foundation

- **Prioritize** foods that are nutrient-rich, satisfying, and help fuel your body for fat loss. Think lean proteins (like chicken, fish, tofu), veggies, whole grains, and healthy fats (avocados, olive oil, nuts). These are the foods that support your goals and keep you full.

- **Enjoy** carbs like sweet potatoes, brown rice, quinoa, and fruits (especially low-sugar ones like berries, apples). These are sources of energy and essential vitamins that keep your body running smoothly.

What About Treats?

Here's the No BS part: you can still enjoy those foods, but let's stop putting them on a pedestal like they're something special. A Snickers bar is just a bunch of sugar and calories in disguise. But if you want one, eat it. Just make a smart trade-off and understand it's no magic food that's going to make or break your results.

- **The Snickers?** Sure, it's sweet and satisfying, but it's just a sugar hit. Want it? Fine, but swap it out for something that will work for your body: **a high-protein bar** with less sugar but still gives you the sweet fix. More protein, fewer empty calories.

- **Regular soda?** Same deal. It's sugar and chemicals. Instead, go for a **Coke Zero**. No calories, same refreshment.

- **Muffins or pastries?** Just more empty calories and sugar. Try **Greek yogurt with a handful of berries**. You'll satisfy your craving with more protein and nutrients.

The Truth About Treats

Here's the deal: Those "special" foods like Snickers, muffins, or sugary drinks are just calories, and most of the time, they're not worth it for fat loss. When you take them off their pedestal, you realize they don't hold the power you think they do.

- **The trick is**: You can still have the Snickers, the muffin, or whatever your treat is—but with awareness. If you've already had 1700 calories for the day and you've got 250 left, go ahead and have the Snickers. But **don't make it your entire day**—balance it out and make it fit.

- **Important**: **Nothing special about the Snickers**—it's just a choice. Treat it like that, and you'll be free to enjoy the foods you like without guilt or overcomplicating things. The key is moderation, portion control, and making it fit with the rest of your goals.

Cheat Days? No Thanks!

I don't support cheat days, plain and simple. Why? Because I believe in eating in a way where cheat days don't even exist. Think about it this way—would you cheat on your spouse? No, you wouldn't. So why cheat on your diet? It's about building a lifestyle where you enjoy what you eat while staying on track.

Here's the truth: People who rely on cheat days often end up sabotaging their progress. Let's break it down. You work your ass off all week, staying in a 2,500-calorie deficit by sticking to your diet and training hard—**WIN!** But then the weekend hits, and you go on a "cheat day." You slurp down 3,500 calories of shitty food in one day, and suddenly your weekly deficit disappears. You're not in a 2,500-calorie deficit anymore. Now, you're in a **1,000-calorie surplus** because of that one binge.

Check the math. You busted your ass all week just to blow it in one day.

Here's what I do instead:

If I want to eat a piece of cake now, I'll eat that damn cake. No cheat day needed.

Let's say that cake was **500 calories**, and my daily calorie needs are **2,800**. Now I have **2,300 calories** left to use for the day. What do I do with those 2,300 calories? Instead of wasting them on more junk, I'll **fuel up with the best**: salads, lean proteins, fruits, and other nutrient-dense foods that will keep me on track.

By adapting and balancing my intake in real time, I can enjoy my cake and still hit my goals. No need to go overboard on a cheat day and blow all my progress.

The No BS Philosophy on Food Choices

Here's the truth: You don't need to cut out the foods you love to lose weight or build muscle. The key isn't about restriction—it's about **smart choices, moderation, and portion control**.

Want a slice of pizza? Eat it. Just be mindful of the portion and how it fits into your day. Want ice cream? Go ahead. But plan for it—know how many calories it'll add, and balance it out with other meals.

It's not about what you can't have—it's about **what you can enjoy** while staying on track. **Flexibility is part of the process**. You can still enjoy your favorite foods as long as they fit into your overall calorie and macronutrient goals.

Now, while treats and cravings are part of life, let's not forget that **the foundation of your diet should still be whole, nutrient-dense foods**. When you focus on nourishing your body with **high-quality foods**, you'll see better results in the long run.

Make every meal count, but remember: **balance and consistency are the keys to lasting success**. Enjoy the foods you love without guilt, and focus on what you can do to stay on track —one meal at a time.

Remember: Your main focus is fat loss, but don't overcomplicate things. If you're craving a Snickers, go ahead and have it. Just keep in mind that a 50g Snickers bar has around 245-250 calories. If you want a lower-calorie option but still want something satisfying, swap it for a high-protein snack, like a protein bar.

Here's the thing: if you've already eaten 1700 calories for the day and you have roughly 245 calories left, then go ahead and enjoy that Snickers, muffin, or whatever else you're craving. It's about fitting it into your daily intake, not depriving yourself. No food is off-limits as long as you're mindful of your goals.

Keep it simple, make smart choices, and stay consistent. Your progress will follow.

3. Meal Ideas for Simplicity and Flexibility

Like we said earlier, we're not diving into full-on recipes here. Instead, the goal is to give you a simple overview of meal ideas that are flexible and adaptable to your needs. Losing weight doesn't mean you're stuck eating bland, overcooked white chicken breast every day. In fact, if that's what comes to your mind when you think about weight loss, we need to change that mindset.

Here are a few ideas that are quick to make, nutrient-packed, and, most importantly, don't taste like cardboard.

Breakfast Options

Starting your day right is crucial for weight loss, and breakfast doesn't have to be boring. I've never been big into breakfasts myself, so I usually just grab a quick 2-scoop protein shake. But for those who enjoy a more substantial meal, here are some simple, flexible ideas that pack a punch without sacrificing flavor:

1. Savory Protein Scramble

- **Overview**: Whip up a quick scramble using eggs or egg whites with spinach, tomatoes, and your choice of lean protein, like turkey or chicken.
- **Why It Works**: This combination is high in protein, keeps you full, and incorporates veggies for added nutrients. Feel free to switch it up with different seasonings or veggies to keep it interesting.

2. Overnight Oats (Customizable!)

- **Overview**: Combine rolled oats with your choice of milk or yogurt, and let them soak overnight. Add fruits, nuts, or seeds in the morning for flavor.
- **Why It Works**: It's a convenient, no-cook option packed with fiber and healthy fats. You can mix and match your toppings to suit your taste.

3. Smoothie Bowl

- **Overview**: Blend your favorite fruits with spinach or kale, and pour it into a bowl. Top with granola, seeds, or nuts.

- **Why It Works**: This is a great way to sneak in some greens while enjoying a refreshing breakfast. You control the ingredients, so it can be tailored to fit your calorie needs.

4. Greek Yogurt Parfait

- **Overview**: Layer plain Greek yogurt with berries, a sprinkle of granola, and a drizzle of honey.
- **Why It Works**: This combination gives you protein, fiber, and a touch of sweetness to kickstart your day without the sugar crash. Adjust the portions based on your calorie goals.

5. Avocado Toast with Eggs

- **Overview**: Smash some avocado on whole-grain toast and top it with a poached or fried egg.
- **Why It Works**: Avocado provides healthy fats, while the egg adds protein, keeping you satisfied until your next meal. You can spice it up with seasonings or hot sauce for extra flavor.

Lunch Options

Lunch is a crucial part of your day, and it should be as easy and enjoyable as possible. Here are some straightforward, nutritious ideas that keep you on track without turning your meal into a chore:

1. Grilled Chicken Salad

- **Overview**: Toss together mixed greens, grilled chicken breast, cherry tomatoes, cucumbers, and your favorite dressing.
- **Why It Works**: Packed with protein and colorful veggies, this salad is filling and refreshing. It's a great way to get your greens in while satisfying your hunger. Plus, it's quick to whip up, making it perfect for those busy days.

2. Wrap It Up

- **Overview**: Use a whole-grain tortilla and fill it with lean protein (like turkey or hummus), mixed greens, and your choice of veggies.
- **Why It Works**: Wraps are portable, easy to make, and can be filled with whatever you like. They're perfect for a quick lunch that keeps you satisfied. Get creative with your fillings—think spicy mustard, avocado, or roasted red peppers to take it up a notch!

3. Stir-Fried Rice or Cauliflower Rice

- **Overview**: Stir-fry brown rice or cauliflower rice with mixed vegetables and a protein source like shrimp or chicken. Add soy sauce or teriyaki for flavor.
- **Why It Works**: This dish is quick, easy, and allows you to clean out your fridge by using up leftover veggies. It's a great way to boost your veggie intake while still enjoying a filling meal. Plus, you can customize it endlessly—add some spice or switch up the protein for variety!

4. Quick and Easy Pizza

- **Overview**: Use a whole-grain pita or tortilla as your base, spread some tomato sauce, and top it with lean protein (like grilled chicken or turkey salami), veggies, and a sprinkle of cheese. Bake or microwave until the cheese is melted.
- **Why It Works**: This is a fun, healthier spin on pizza that satisfies those cravings without derailing your goals. Turkey salami adds a delicious, savory flavor that elevates the whole dish. You get to customize it with your favorite toppings, making it a perfect way to enjoy a classic comfort food.

5. Taco Salad

- **Overview**: Layer a bowl with mixed greens, seasoned ground turkey or beef, black beans, corn, diced tomatoes, and a dollop of Greek yogurt or avocado instead of sour cream.
- **Why It Works**: This dish combines the flavors of tacos without the carbs of tortillas. It's colorful, filling, and packed with protein and fiber. You can adjust the spices and toppings to fit your taste, and it's perfect for meal prep!

Snack Options

Snacking can be a key part of your weight loss journey, helping to curb cravings and keep your energy levels up throughout the day. Here are some easy, satisfying, and fun snack ideas that align with your goals:

1. Protein Bars

- **Overview**: Choose bars that are low in sugar and high in protein. Look for ones made with whole ingredients for a nutritious boost.
- **Why It Works**: Protein bars are convenient and perfect for on-the-go snacking. They help you meet your protein goals without much effort and come in a variety of flavors, making them a tasty treat.

2. Protein Shakes

- **Overview**: Blend your favorite protein powder with water or milk, and consider adding fruits like bananas or berries for extra flavor and nutrients.
- **Why It Works**: Protein shakes are quick and easy, especially after workouts. They can also be customized with fun additions like nut butter, spinach, or cocoa powder for a delicious and filling snack.

3. Fresh Fruits

- **Overview**: Stock up on a variety of fruits like apples, bananas, berries, and oranges for a refreshing and nutritious snack.
- **Why It Works**: Fruits are naturally sweet and hydrating. They can be made more fun by slicing them up and creating fruit skewers, or pairing them with yogurt or a drizzle of honey.

4. Mixed Nuts

- **Overview**: A handful of assorted nuts like almonds, walnuts, or cashews makes for a great snack.
- **Why It Works**: Nuts are a source of healthy fats, protein, and fiber. To make it more fun, consider creating your own trail mix by combining nuts with dried fruits, seeds, and a sprinkle of dark chocolate chips.

5. Veggies with Hummus

- **Overview**: Pair crunchy veggies like carrots, celery, and bell peppers with a serving of hummus for dipping.
- **Why It Works**: This combo is low in calories but high in nutrients. To make it more enjoyable, try creating a veggie platter for a mini party, mixing in some colorful dips like guacamole or tzatziki.

6. Popcorn

- **Overview**: Air-popped popcorn is a great low-calorie snack that you can season however you like.
- **Why It Works**: It's fun to experiment with flavors—try sprinkling it with nutritional yeast for a cheesy taste, or adding a dash of cinnamon for a sweet twist. Plus, it's light and satisfying, making it perfect for movie nights!

7. Yogurt Parfaits

- **Overview**: Layer Greek yogurt with fresh fruits and a sprinkle of granola or nuts.
- **Why It Works**: Yogurt parfaits are not only delicious but also visually appealing. They can be customized to your taste and are perfect for breakfast or a snack. Mix and match fruits and toppings for variety!

Dinner Options

Dinner is a great opportunity to refuel after a long day, and it doesn't have to be complicated. Here are some easy and satisfying dinner ideas that fit your goals and tastes:

1. Spaghetti Bolognese

- **Overview**: Prepare a classic Bolognese sauce using only minced meat, tomatoes, garlic, and your choice of herbs. Serve it over whole-grain spaghetti or zucchini noodles for a healthier twist.
- **Why It Works**: This dish is hearty and filling, making it a perfect comfort food. By using minced meat, you keep it simple while still getting a good protein source. It's also easy to make in larger batches, allowing for leftovers or meal prep.

2. Stir-Fried Chicken and Vegetables

- **Overview**: Toss together diced chicken breast with a variety of colorful veggies like bell peppers, broccoli, and carrots. Add some soy sauce or teriyaki for flavor and serve over brown rice or quinoa.
- **Why It Works**: This dish is quick to prepare and can be customized based on what veggies you have on hand. It's a great way to pack in lean protein and fiber-rich vegetables, keeping your dinner nutritious and satisfying.

3. Grilled Salmon with Asparagus

- **Overview**: Season a salmon fillet with lemon, garlic, and herbs, then grill it alongside fresh asparagus. Serve with a side of quinoa or a simple salad.
- **Why It Works**: Salmon is rich in omega-3 fatty acids and protein, making it a heart-healthy choice. Asparagus adds vitamins and minerals, while the quinoa provides a good source of complex carbohydrates.

4. Taco Night

- **Overview**: Use lean ground turkey or beef for your tacos, and fill corn or whole-grain tortillas with your favorite toppings like lettuce, tomatoes, salsa, and avocado.
- **Why It Works**: Taco night is fun and allows for creativity in the kitchen. You can customize each taco to your liking, making it a crowd-pleaser. Plus, it's a great way to incorporate more veggies into your meal!

5. Baked Sweet Potato with Toppings

- **Overview**: Bake sweet potatoes until tender and top them with a mix of Greek yogurt, black beans, salsa, and a sprinkle of cheese or avocado.
- **Why It Works**: This dish is simple, hearty, and full of flavor. Sweet potatoes are a fantastic source of complex carbs and fiber, and adding toppings keeps it interesting. It's a versatile meal that can easily adapt to your tastes!

Final Thoughts on Meal Ideas

Remember, weight loss doesn't have to mean sacrificing flavor or settling for boring meals. The key is to get creative and enjoy the foods you love while still achieving your goals. Eating should be an enjoyable experience, not a chore.

So, as you plan your meals, focus on variety and excitement. By incorporating delicious options like those we've discussed, you can keep your meals vibrant, satisfying, and far from bland. After all, who wants to eat dry, overcooked chicken when you can whip up something tasty and fulfilling?

And here's the kicker:

If you've nailed your nutrition for the day and find yourself with 300 calories left, don't hesitate—grab that doughnut! Treat it as a reward for all your hard work. You've earned it! No bullshit.

Embrace the idea that healthy eating can be delicious, fun, and still leave room for treats.

Real-Life Adaptation: Flexibility is Key

The No BS Diet isn't about eliminating foods or sticking to a restrictive meal plan. It's about making smarter choices in real-life situations while enjoying the foods you love. Flexibility is essential to achieving sustainable results.

1. Making Smart Choices: Navigating Food and Drink in Everyday Life

Eating Out

Don't stress about every single meal when dining out. Instead, focus on making healthier choices. Look for options like grilled, baked, or steamed dishes. For instance, swap out fries for a side salad or steamed veggies, and ask for dressings on the side to control how much you use. Enjoying a meal out should be a pleasure, not a source of anxiety.

Social Situations

Heading to a party? It's perfectly okay to indulge in a piece of cake or a slice of pizza. The key is to make good decisions most of the time without obsessing over the occasional treat. You don't have to be perfect to see results—consistency and balance are what truly matter. Enjoying food in social settings can enhance your experience and help you build lasting habits.

Mindful Eating

Practice mindful eating by savoring your food, paying attention to your hunger and fullness cues, and truly enjoying each bite. This can help reduce overeating and increase satisfaction with your meals.

Meal Prep and Planning

Rather than strict meal prepping, I focused on making meals exciting and intuitive. I allowed myself to decide what I felt like eating each day, which made the process enjoyable. The only planning I did involved getting rid of unhealthy items and swapping them out for better alternatives. This approach made it much harder to choose something unhealthy when it came time to prepare lunch or dinner. When your environment supports your goals, making the right choices becomes second nature.

Embrace Imperfection

Remember, nobody is perfect, and it's okay to have off days. If you indulge in something less healthy, enjoy it without guilt. Just don't go overboard. It's all part of the process, and balance is key.

Nighttime Hunger Struggles

I know firsthand how challenging nighttime cravings can be. There were nights when I'd hear my stomach growling, battling that relentless voice in my head urging me to snack. It's essential to recognize these feelings and understand that it's normal to experience hunger at night. Instead of succumbing to mindless snacking, try to have a plan in place for healthy options that satisfy your cravings without derailing your progress.

Portion Control

When enjoying your favorite foods, be mindful of portion sizes. This way, you can savor the flavors without going overboard.

Hydration and Healthy Snacks

Stay hydrated and keep healthy snacks on hand. This can help manage hunger and prevent impulsive, unhealthy choices when you're busy or on the go.

2. Alcohol Awareness: Understanding Your Choices

Many people underestimate the number of calories in alcoholic beverages, which can significantly impact your progress. Here's what you need to know:

- **Mind the Calories**: Alcohol can be surprisingly calorie-dense. For instance, a standard beer can contain around 150 calories, while a glass of wine may have about 120-150 calories. Cocktails, especially those made with sugary mixers, can have even more, sometimes exceeding 500 calories for just one drink.

- **Choose Wisely**: Opt for lighter options when drinking. A glass of wine or spirits with zero-calorie mixers (like soda water) can be a better choice than high-calorie cocktails. Being mindful of what you drink can help you enjoy your social life without derailing your goals.

- **Moderation is Key**: It's perfectly fine to enjoy a drink or two, but be aware of how they fit into your overall calorie intake for the day. If you know you're going to indulge in alcohol, plan your other meals accordingly to maintain a balance.

- **Balance is Crucial**: Enjoying alcohol doesn't have to mean giving up on your goals. The key is to enjoy it in moderation, ensuring it doesn't become a regular source of excessive calories.

By being aware of the calories in alcohol and making smarter choices, you can still enjoy your social life while staying on track with your goals.

Low-Calorie Drink Recommendations

1. **Wine:**

   o **Dry Red or White Wine:** Approximately 120-150 calories per 5 oz. glass. Look for dry varieties as they tend to have lower sugar content.

2. **Light Beer:**

   o **Light Beer:** Typically around 90-110 calories per 12 oz. serving. These beers are brewed to have fewer calories than regular beers.

3. **Spirits with Zero-Calorie Mixers:**

   o **Vodka Soda:** Mix 1.5 oz. of vodka with soda water and a squeeze of lime. Approximately 100 calories.

   o **Gin and Tonic (with Diet Tonic):** Use diet tonic water to cut calories to around 100-120 for a standard drink.

   o **Rum and Diet Coke:** Combine 1.5 oz. of rum with diet cola for a refreshing drink that's around 100 calories.

4. **Hard Seltzers:**

   o **Hard Seltzers:** Generally range from 80-100 calories per 12 oz. can, making them a light and refreshing option.

5. **Sparkling Water with a Splash of Juice:**

   o **Sparkling Water:** Mix with a splash (about 1 oz.) of your favorite juice for a flavorful drink while keeping calories low. This can be around 20-50 calories depending on the juice.

6. **Infused Water or Herbal Tea:**

   o While not alcoholic, offering **infused water** (water with slices of fruit, cucumber, or herbs) or **herbal tea** can be a great non-alcoholic alternative for social occasions. They have negligible calories and are refreshing.

7. **Low-Calorie Cocktails:**

   o **Skinny Margarita:** Use 1.5 oz. tequila, 1 oz. lime juice, and 1 oz. soda water for a lighter version, around 150 calories.

   o **Mojito (without sugar):** Muddle mint leaves and lime juice, add 1.5 oz. rum and soda water for a refreshing drink, around 100 calories.

Summary

When making choices about drinks, remember to enjoy them in moderation while being mindful of their caloric content. By opting for these low-calorie options, you can enjoy social gatherings without compromising your weight loss efforts.

Focus on Sustainable Habits (Not Perfection)

The most crucial aspect of the No BS Diet is sustainability. Drastic, short-term measures won't help you lose weight in the long run, and often they lead to burnout or yo-yo dieting. Instead, the key is to build habits that last a lifetime, ensuring you see results that you can maintain.

Embrace Progress Over Perfection

You don't need to eat chicken and broccoli every day, nor do you have to skip your favorite foods entirely. Real progress comes from making consistent, healthier choices over time. The occasional indulgence isn't going to ruin your efforts—what matters is what you do most of the time, not all the time. Focus on progress rather than striving for unrealistic perfection. A slip-up here and there is normal, and it's how you recover from those moments that truly matters.

The Power of Sustainable Choices

Incorporating healthier choices into your routine doesn't have to mean giving up the foods you love. It's about making small, smart swaps—choosing grilled chicken over fried, adding more veggies to your meals, or having water instead of sugary drinks. These simple choices may seem insignificant at first, but over time, they compound and lead to real, lasting results. The key is making decisions you can stick with for the long haul, not just during a "diet phase."

Build Habits Gradually

It's tempting to overhaul your entire diet and exercise plan overnight, but drastic changes are rarely sustainable. Instead, focus on building new habits gradually. Start with one or two small goals—like eating a protein-packed breakfast or going for a daily walk—and once those become second nature, add more. This approach reduces the feeling of overwhelm and helps make the changes a permanent part of your lifestyle.

Celebrate the Small Wins

Often, people get caught up in the bigger picture and overlook the small victories along the way. Did you skip dessert for a healthier option today? Did you get a workout in even though you were tired? These are wins! Acknowledge them, because they reflect the gradual progress that leads to long-term success. Don't wait for the end goal to celebrate—appreciate every step you take toward it.

Plan for Flexibility

Sustainability requires flexibility. Life will always throw curveballs—unexpected events, social gatherings, busy days, and stressful situations. Rather than getting derailed by these, allow room for adjustments. If you overindulge at a meal, balance it out by making a healthier choice at the next one. If you miss a workout, don't beat yourself up—get back on track tomorrow. The key is to develop resilience and adaptability, not rigidity.

Sustainable Habits Over Fad Diets

Fad diets might promise quick results, but they're often too restrictive and unsustainable. Instead of cutting out entire food groups or following extreme regimens, focus on balance and moderation. Incorporate whole foods like lean proteins, vegetables, fruits, and whole grains into your meals while allowing room for the occasional indulgence. This balance keeps you from feeling deprived and ensures that your weight loss journey is enjoyable, not a constant struggle.

Make It Enjoyable

If you dread your meals or your workout routine, you won't stick with them for long. Find ways to make your diet and exercise plan enjoyable. Experiment with new recipes, find a workout you love, or set goals that keep you motivated. When you enjoy what you're doing, it becomes easier to maintain those habits over time.

Remember: Results Take Time

We all want fast results, but the reality is that the best kind of weight loss is gradual and steady. Fad diets and extreme restrictions might deliver quick changes, but those results are rarely sustainable. What you're aiming for isn't just a number on the scale—it's lasting change, healthier habits, and a body that feels strong and energized.

Focus on Small, Consistent Changes

Instead of chasing quick fixes, focus on the small changes you can make day by day. It's these consistent actions that compound over time and create sustainable habits. You might not notice dramatic shifts overnight, but if you stay patient and trust the process, you'll wake up one day and realize just how far you've come.

Guaranteed Results (With Consistency)

If you follow the principles outlined in this chapter, I guarantee you'll lose weight. This isn't a crash diet that leaves you feeling miserable or deprived. It's about eating real, nutritious food in the right balance while staying consistent with your choices. By creating sustainable habits, you'll not only lose weight—you'll keep it off. The focus is on living a healthy life that you can enjoy, without constantly feeling restricted or hungry.

Trust the Process

Results might not come as quickly as you want, and that's okay. Trust the process and believe in your ability to make lasting change. Keep reminding yourself that it's not a race—it's about long-term success. Every step, no matter how small, moves you closer to your goals. As you progress, your mindset will shift, and these healthier habits will become part of your daily routine.

Next Steps: Preparing for Fitness

In the upcoming chapters, I'll dive deeper into workout plans, cardio strategies, and strength training routines that will help you burn fat faster and preserve muscle. But for now, your focus should be on getting your nutrition right. When you build balanced meals and practice consistency with your food choices, your body composition will start to shift. You'll be laying the foundation for a stronger, leaner body, primed for the physical challenges ahead.

No Bullshit Diet = Real Results

There you have it—the No BS Diet. It's not complicated, it's not restrictive, and it doesn't require extreme sacrifices. The key is making smart, consistent choices by focusing on nutrient-dense, whole foods most of the time. No gimmicks, no tricks—just real, sustainable habits that deliver real results.

You've got everything you need to lose fat, build muscle, and get the body you want. Now it's time to take action and put these principles into practice.

Let's get to work.

Chapter 3: Workout Plans: Build Muscle, Get Healthier, Boost Fat Loss

I. Introduction

In this chapter, we'll dive into practical workout plans designed to build muscle, improve overall health, and support fat loss. The routines you'll find here are straightforward yet effective, aiming to deliver real results without the fluff. Whether you're new to the gym or have been lifting for years, these plans are adaptable to fit your current fitness level while offering a clear path for progression.

One of the key principles you'll discover is that your gym routine is more than just a physical activity—it's a powerful tool for transforming your body. Beyond aesthetics, these workouts help improve cardiovascular health, increase metabolism, and promote mental well-being. Consistency in your gym routine will not only lead to fat loss but also create long-term habits for a healthier lifestyle.

To achieve the best results, it's essential to strike a balance between strength training and cardio. Strength training builds lean muscle, which increases your resting metabolic rate—meaning your body burns more calories, even when you're not working out. On the other hand, cardio enhances heart health and helps burn extra calories in the short term. Together, these elements create a comprehensive fitness plan that targets multiple aspects of health, ensuring you're not just getting leaner but also stronger and fitter over time. That being said, I strongly recommend this lifestyle—not just for fat loss, but for everything that comes with working out: better health, more energy, improved muscle tone, and stronger mental resilience. Regular workouts don't just change how you look, but how you feel—more confident, focused, and driven.

However, in keeping with the no-nonsense approach of this book, let me be clear: **you don't have to work out to lose weight**. If your only goal is weight loss and you don't feel like hitting the gym, that's completely your choice. As I've explained earlier, weight loss is all about eating in a calorie deficit. If working out isn't your thing, go back to the nutrition and mindset sections and get started from there.

That said, here's the truth: **working out will speed up the process considerably**. Strength training builds muscle, which burns more calories even when you're at rest. Cardio boosts your calorie burn and improves overall heart health. Combining these will help you not only lose weight faster but also ensure you maintain muscle mass and get healthier as you go. The choice is yours, but if you're looking for maximum results, the workouts in this chapter will get you there faster.

Strength Training Basics for Fat Loss

Why Strength Training Matters

Strength training is a critical component of any effective workout plan, especially for fat loss. When you build muscle, you're not just enhancing your physique; you're also revving up your metabolism. Muscle tissue is metabolically active, meaning it requires more energy (calories) to maintain than fat tissue. In simple terms, the more muscle you have, the more calories you burn at rest. This increased resting metabolic rate can lead to greater fat loss over time, even when you're not in the gym.

Moreover, strength training fosters discipline. When you commit to a workout routine, you're investing not only your time and effort but also your hard-earned money into your gym membership. This investment can create a mental framework that reinforces healthy eating habits. Knowing you've worked hard in the gym makes it easier to resist temptations and stick to your diet. After all, it's much harder to justify junk food when you visualize the sweat and determination that went into your workouts. This mindset creates a powerful cycle of accountability, helping you stay on track toward your goals.

Myth-Busting: Lifting Weights Won't Make You "Bulky" (Revised)

A common misconception is that lifting weights will make you bulky, especially among women. This myth stems from the idea that all strength training leads to excessive muscle gain. In reality, building significant muscle mass takes multiple years of consistent training, proper nutrition, and dedication.

It took me 10 years to reach the physique I have today, and I can assure you it is nowhere near what most would define as bulky. My experience illustrates that, for most people focused on fat loss and overall fitness, strength training will lead to a toned and lean appearance rather than excess bulk.

In bodybuilding and powerlifting, there's a term called "bulking." This refers to eating in a caloric surplus while training hard to accelerate muscle gain. After this phase, many individuals enter a "cut" phase, where they focus on losing fat to reveal their muscle gains.

For those of us training diligently and focusing on a balanced approach, strength training promotes a fit and athletic look. You can achieve a well-defined physique through consistent effort in the gym and smart nutritional choices without the risk of becoming excessively bulky.

Key Strength Training Principles

Compound vs. Isolation Movements

When designing your workout routine, it's essential to understand the difference between compound and isolation movements.

Compound Movements: These exercises involve multiple muscle groups and joints, making them highly effective for building strength and muscle. They are particularly beneficial for fat loss due to their higher calorie expenditure. Here are some examples of key compound movements:

- **Squats**: Targeting your quads, hamstrings, glutes, and core, squats improve lower body strength and stability. Aim for proper form by keeping your chest up and your knees aligned with your toes.

- **Deadlifts**: Engaging your back, glutes, hamstrings, and core, deadlifts promote overall strength. Ensure your back is straight and your hips drive forward to lift the weight effectively.

- **Bench Press**: Primarily working the chest, shoulders, and triceps, this exercise builds upper body strength. Keep your feet flat on the ground and your elbows at a 45-degree angle during the lift.

- **Military Press**: This overhead press targets the shoulders, triceps, and upper chest, helping to build upper body strength and stability. Maintain a strong core and avoid arching your back during the lift.

While these are just a few examples of compound movements, prioritizing them in your routine will yield better results for overall fitness and fat loss. Their higher calorie expenditure and greater muscle recruitment make them a cornerstone of an effective workout plan.

Isolation Movements: These exercises focus on a single muscle group and are great for targeting specific areas. Examples include:

- **Bicep Curls**: Primarily targeting the biceps, this exercise helps to build arm strength and size.

- **Tricep Extensions**: Focusing on the triceps, this movement enhances the overall definition of the upper arms.

- **Lateral Raises**: This exercise targets the shoulders, helping to build width and definition in the upper body.

- **Leg Curls**: Isolating the hamstrings, leg curls are effective for strengthening the back of the thighs.

While isolation exercises can be useful, especially for refining muscle definition, they generally burn fewer calories compared to compound movements. Thus, incorporating a mix of both types of exercises will help you achieve a balanced and effective workout routine.

Key Strength Training Principles

Progressive Overload

To achieve continuous results in your strength training, it's essential to implement the principle of **progressive overload**. This means gradually increasing the demands placed on your muscles to stimulate growth and adaptation. Here's how you can effectively apply progressive overload in your workouts:

- **Increase Weights**: Aim to lift heavier weights over time as your strength improves. Small increments (e.g., 2.5 to 5 pounds) can make a significant difference when you're consistently challenging yourself.

- **Increase Reps**: If you can comfortably complete your sets with good form, consider adding more repetitions. For example, if you're doing 3 sets of 10 reps, try increasing to 3 sets of 12 reps before adding weight.

- **Increase Sets**: Adding more sets to your workout can also increase total volume and intensity. If you usually do 3 sets of an exercise, try increasing to 4 or 5 sets for additional challenge.

- **Change Tempo**: Slowing down the eccentric (lowering) phase of an exercise can increase tension on the muscles and promote growth. For instance, take 3-4 seconds to lower the weight during a squat instead of a quick drop.

- **Push Yourself**: It's essential to push yourself during each exercise to maximize your results. Rather than aiming for the same number of reps with the same weight across all sets, consider structuring your sets like this:

Understanding How to Push Yourself During Workouts

To achieve continuous growth and improvement, it's essential to learn how to push yourself effectively. This doesn't mean maxing out on every set, but instead knowing how to manage your effort across multiple sets to maximize gains while maintaining form and minimizing the risk of injury.

In the example provided, you can see how to exert yourself across different sets:

Set 1: 12 reps (leaving 1-2 reps in reserve)
You start with a weight that allows you to complete 12 repetitions comfortably. By leaving 1-2 reps in reserve, you're building a strong foundation for the following sets without exhausting yourself immediately.

Set 2: 11 reps (leaving 1-2 reps in reserve again)
The second set becomes more challenging as your muscles begin to tire, but you still maintain control and leave a couple of reps in reserve. This helps you maintain good form and prepares you for greater exertion in subsequent sets.

Set 3: 9 reps (leaving 1 rep in reserve)
In this set, you push yourself further. Completing 9 reps while leaving only 1 rep in reserve means you're nearing your limit, feeling the burn, and pushing your muscles to adapt.

Set 4: 8 reps (pushing to failure)
In the final set, you push yourself to failure, completing 8 reps and fully engaging your muscles. This is where you maximize effort and stimulate growth as your muscles are forced to adapt to the challenge.

Highlight: If you notice that your rep progression from set one to set four is decreasing, it's a clear indicator that you're pushing yourself. This natural drop in reps shows that your muscles are becoming fatigued, which means you're exerting yourself effectively and promoting muscle growth and adaptation.

Why It Matters

By using this method of progressive overload, you ensure that you're consistently challenging your body. This strategy prevents plateaus—where you stop seeing progress—by keeping your muscles guessing. Each set requires more effort, pushing you to improve both strength and endurance over time.

Incorporating progressive overload into your workouts builds discipline, as you'll feel more accountable for pushing yourself each session. You're not just going through the motions; you're actively seeking to improve, making it harder to stray from your diet and fitness goals. This approach fosters a mindset of growth, helping you to become not only physically stronger but also mentally tougher in your journey toward your fitness aspirations.

The Problem with Doing the Same 4 Sets of 12 Reps

Let's be real—if you're walking into the gym and doing the same 4 sets of exactly 12 reps with the same weight every single time, you're not really doing much. Sure, you're moving, but your body isn't being pushed to adapt or change. Here's why:

1. **Zero Progress:** By sticking to the same weight and reps, you're just maintaining the status quo. You're not forcing your muscles to grow or get stronger because they're not being challenged. So, don't be surprised if after months of doing this, your body looks exactly the same.

2. **No Adaptation:** Your muscles only grow when they're given a reason to. If you're lifting the same weight for the same reps every session, you're telling your muscles they're already good enough. No growth, no fat loss—just staying in the same place.

3. **Wasting Time:** Let's be blunt—going through the motions without pushing yourself is just wasting time. If you're going to be in the gym, make it count. You might as well push yourself hard and see real results instead of just spinning your wheels.

In contrast, using progressive overload like we discussed earlier—pushing for fewer reps as you fatigue, lifting heavier over time—forces your body to adapt. That's how you break through plateaus and actually see the changes you're working for.

This approach shows that you're actively challenging your muscles as you progress through your sets. Even if you've been working out for years, incorporating this level of effort and structure can lead to significant changes. Consistently pushing your limits is key to overcoming plateaus and continuing to make progress in your strength training journey.

Rest Periods and Intensity

Why Shorter Rest Periods Burn More Calories

Rest periods are crucial to how effective your workout is for fat loss. Shorter rest periods (30-60 seconds) between sets help keep your heart rate elevated, leading to higher calorie burn. This approach not only boosts cardiovascular fitness but also improves metabolic efficiency, allowing your body to continue burning calories even after your workout ends.

Using Supersets and Circuit Training to Elevate Heart Rate

Supersets and circuit training are great strategies to push your intensity and elevate your heart rate:

- **Supersets:** Pair two exercises back-to-back without resting in between. For instance, you could do a triceps extensions followed immediately by lateral raises, keeping intensity high and burning more calories in a shorter time.

- **Circuit Training:** Rotate through multiple exercises with little rest. A typical circuit could include squats, kettlebell swings, push-ups, and planks, targeting different muscle groups to sustain your heart rate and maximize fat loss.

When to Use Longer Rest Periods

For compound movements that focus on building pure strength, such as squats, deadlifts, and military presses, longer rest periods (2-3 minutes) are often necessary. These exercises are more taxing on your body, requiring additional recovery time between sets to maintain good form and maximize strength output.

Balancing both shorter rest for fat loss and longer rest for strength-focused compound movements will give you the best of both worlds—burning fat while building strength effectively.

Sample Strength Training Workouts

Workout Programs:

1. **Full-Body Routine (3x per week)**
   This program focuses on working all major muscle groups in a single session. Ideal for beginners and those short on time, it emphasizes functional, compound movements like squats, deadlifts, and bench presses.

Workout A:

- **Squats** – 4 sets x 8-10 reps
  Target: Quads, hamstrings, glutes, core
- **Bench Press** – 4 sets x 8-10 reps
  Target: Chest, shoulders, triceps
- **Bent Over Rows** – 4 sets x 8-10 reps
  Target: Back, biceps, rear delts
- **Overhead Press** – 3 sets x 8-10 reps
  Target: Shoulders, triceps
- **Triceps Extensions** – 3 sets x 10-12 reps
  Target: Triceps
- **Plank** – 3 sets of 30-60 seconds
  Target: Core

Workout B:

- **Deadlifts** – 4 sets x 6-8 reps
  Target: Hamstrings, glutes, lower back
- **Pull-Ups (or Lat Pulldowns)** – 4 sets x 8-10 reps
  Target: Back, biceps
- **Dumbbell Lunges** – 4 sets x 10 reps per leg
  Target: Quads, glutes, hamstrings
- **Incline Dumbbell Press** – 4 sets x 8-10 reps
  Target: Chest, shoulders, triceps

* **Leg Press** – 3 sets x 10-12 reps
  Target: Quads, hamstrings, glutes
* **Bicep Curls** – 3 sets x 10-12 reps
  Target: Biceps
* **Russian Twists** – 3 sets x 20 reps per side
  Target: Core

Guidelines:

* **Rest Periods**: 60-90 seconds between sets.
* **Frequency**: Perform this routine 3x per week (e.g., Monday, Wednesday, Friday) with at least one day of rest between sessions.
* **Progressive Overload**: Each week, aim to increase the weight or reps as you build strength.
* **Cardio**: Optional—add 20-30 minutes of moderate-intensity cardio at the end for additional fat loss.

Weekly Routine Split:

* **Week 1**: Workout A | Workout B | Workout A
* **Week 2**: Workout B | Workout A | Workout B

This setup ensures you work all major muscle groups evenly, avoid overtraining, and allow for optimal recovery between sessions.

2. **Upper/Lower Split**

   This split divides your workouts into upper-body and lower-body days, allowing you to train each area twice a week. It's great for those who want more focus on each muscle group without spending too much time in the gym daily.

   * **Frequency:** Train 4 days per week (e.g., Upper A, Lower A, Upper B, Lower B).

Upper Body Workout A

- **Bench Press** – 4 sets x 8-10 reps
  Target: Chest, shoulders, triceps

- **Bent-Over Rows** – 4 sets x 8-10 reps
  Target: Back, biceps, rear delts

- **Overhead Press** – 3 sets x 8-10 reps
  Target: Shoulders, triceps

- **Tricep Dips** – 3 sets x 10-12 reps
  Target: Triceps

- **Face Pulls** – 3 sets x 12-15 reps
  Target: Rear delts, upper back

Lower Body Workout A

- **Deadlifts** – 4 sets x 6-8 reps
  Target: Hamstrings, glutes, lower back

- **Leg Press** – 4 sets x 8-10 reps
  Target: Quads, hamstrings, glutes

- **Leg Curls** – 3 sets x 10-12 reps
  Target: Hamstrings

- **Calf Raises** – 3 sets x 12-15 reps
  Target: Calves

- **Plank** – 3 sets of 30-60 seconds
  Target: Core

Upper Body Workout B

- **Incline Dumbbell Press** – 4 sets x 8-10 reps
  Target: Chest, shoulders, triceps

- **Pull-Ups (or Lat Pulldowns)** – 4 sets x 8-10 reps
  Target: Back, biceps

- **Dumbbell Shoulder Press** – 3 sets x 8-10 reps
  Target: Shoulders, triceps

- **Bicep Curls** – 3 sets x 10-12 reps
  Target: Biceps

- **Dumbbell Lateral Raises** – 3 sets x 12-15 reps
  Target: Shoulders

Lower Body Workout B

- **Squats** – 4 sets x 8-10 reps
  Target: Quads, hamstrings, glutes

- **Dumbbell Lunges** – 4 sets x 10 reps per leg
  Target: Quads, glutes, hamstrings

- **Leg Extensions** – 3 sets x 10-12 reps
  Target: Quads

- **Calf Raises** – 3 sets x 12-15 reps
  Target: Calves

- **Russian Twists** – 3 sets x 20 reps per side
  Target: Core

Guidelines:

- **Rest Periods:** 60-90 seconds between sets.
- **Frequency:** Perform this routine 4x per week (e.g., Monday: Upper A, Tuesday: Lower A, Thursday: Upper B, Friday: Lower B).

- **Progressive Overload:** Each week, aim to increase the weight or reps as you build strength.

This setup allows for a balanced focus on both upper and lower body while maximizing muscle engagement and recovery time.

3. **Push/Pull/Legs (PPL) Split**

   A well-rounded routine where each day is dedicated to pushing movements (like bench presses), pulling movements (like rows), and legs. It provides a balance between strength and hypertrophy, with flexibility to adjust intensity for fat loss.

Push Day (Chest, Shoulders, Triceps)

- **Bench Press** – 4 sets x 8-10 reps
  Target: Chest, shoulders, triceps

- **Overhead Press** – 4 sets x 8-10 reps
  Target: Shoulders, triceps

- **Incline Dumbbell Press** – 3 sets x 8-10 reps
  Target: Upper chest, shoulders, triceps

- **Lateral Raises** – 3 sets x 12-15 reps
  Target: Shoulders

- **Tricep Dips** – 3 sets x 10-12 reps
  Target: Triceps

Pull Day (Back, Biceps)

- **Deadlifts** – 4 sets x 6-8 reps
  Target: Hamstrings, glutes, lower back

- **Pull-Ups (or Lat Pulldowns)** – 4 sets x 8-10 reps
  Target: Back, biceps

- **Barbell Rows** – 4 sets x 8-10 reps
  Target: Back, rear delts

- **Face Pulls** – 3 sets x 12-15 reps
  Target: Upper back, rear delts

- **Bicep Curls** – 3 sets x 10-12 reps
  Target: Biceps

Leg Day (Quads, Hamstrings, Glutes)

- **Squats** – 4 sets x 8-10 reps
  Target: Quads, hamstrings, glutes

- **Leg Press** – 4 sets x 8-10 reps
  Target: Quads, hamstrings

- **Romanian Deadlifts** – 3 sets x 8-10 reps
  Target: Hamstrings, glutes

- **Leg Curls** – 3 sets x 10-12 reps
  Target: Hamstrings

- **Calf Raises** – 3 sets x 12-15 reps
  Target: Calves

Guidelines:

- **Rest Periods:** 60-90 seconds between sets.

- **Frequency:** Ideally performed 6x per week (e.g., Monday: Push, Tuesday: Pull, Wednesday: Legs, Thursday: Push, Friday: Pull, Saturday: Legs), with Sunday as a rest day. *(6 times a week is advanced)*
  Alternatively:

  - **3x per week:** Cycle through Push, Pull, and Legs (e.g., Week 1: Push, Pull, Legs; Week 2: Push, Pull, Legs).
  - **4x per week:** Rotate as Push, Pull, Legs, rest, and then continue (e.g., Monday: Push, Tuesday: Pull, Thursday: Legs, Friday: Push, and so on).

- **Progressive Overload:** Each week, aim to increase the weight or reps as you build strength.

- **Warm-Up**: Begin each session with 5-10 minutes of light cardio and dynamic stretching to prepare your muscles and joints.

- **Recovery**: Ensure adequate rest and sleep for optimal muscle repair and growth between sessions.

4. Calisthenics Routine

Bodyweight-focused exercises such as push-ups, pull-ups, dips, and squats. This program is perfect for people who prefer minimal equipment or want to work on functional strength while losing fat.

Workout A:

1. **Push-Ups** – 4 sets x 10-15 reps
   Target: Chest, shoulders, triceps
2. **Pull-Ups (or Inverted Rows)** – 4 sets x 8-12 reps
   Target: Back, biceps
3. **Bodyweight Squats** – 4 sets x 15-20 reps
   Target: Quads, hamstrings, glutes
4. **Dips (Parallel Bars or Bench Dips)** – 4 sets x 10-12 reps
   Target: Chest, shoulders, triceps
5. **Plank** – 3 sets of 30-60 seconds
   Target: Core
6. **Lunges** – 3 sets x 10 reps per leg
   Target: Quads, hamstrings, glutes

Workout B:

1. **Pike Push-Ups** – 4 sets x 8-12 reps
   Target: Shoulders, triceps
2. **Chin-Ups** – 4 sets x 8-10 reps
   Target: Back, biceps

3. **Bulgarian Split Squats** – 4 sets x 10 reps per leg
   Target: Quads, hamstrings, glutes
4. **Glute Bridges** – 4 sets x 12-15 reps
   Target: Glutes, hamstrings, lower back
5. **Hollow Body Hold** – 3 sets of 30-60 seconds
   Target: Core
6. **Mountain Climbers** – 3 sets of 20 reps per side
   Target: Core, shoulders, legs

Guidelines:

- **Rest Periods**: 45-60 seconds between sets.
- **Frequency**: Perform 3-4x per week (e.g., alternating Workout A and Workout B).
- **Progressive Overload**: Increase reps or add variations (e.g., weighted vests, decline push-ups) as you get stronger.
- **Cardio**: Optional – add short bursts of cardio like jumping jacks or burpees between sets for additional fat loss.

Maximizing Your Workout: Warm-Ups, Split Rotation, Rest, and Recovery

Warm-Ups: Preparing Your Body for Success

A proper warm-up is critical for preparing your muscles, joints, and cardiovascular system for the workout ahead. It reduces the risk of injury and enhances performance.

1. **General Warm-Up** (5-10 minutes): Start with light cardio to get your blood flowing. Choose activities like jogging, cycling, or brisk walking. This raises your heart rate and prepares your body for more intense movements.

2. **Dynamic Stretching & Mobility** (5-10 minutes): Follow up with dynamic stretches targeting the areas you'll work out.

   - **Leg Swings**
   - **Arm Circles**
   - **Hip Rotations**

- o   **Lunges with a Twist** This boosts flexibility and improves your range of motion, priming your body for both compound and isolation exercises.

Split Rotation: Organizing Your Workouts

Each workout split (Full Body, Upper/Lower, PPL, Calisthenics) comes with different rotation structures depending on the frequency of your training. Here's how to schedule them:

- **Full-Body Split** (3x per week): Rotate between **Workout A** and **Workout B** every other session.

  - o   **Week 1:** Monday (A), Wednesday (B), Friday (A)
  - o   **Week 2:** Monday (B), Wednesday (A), Friday (B)
- **Upper/Lower Split** (4x per week): Train the upper and lower body on separate days, alternating through the week.

  - o   **Monday:** Upper
  - o   **Tuesday:** Lower
  - o   **Thursday:** Upper
  - o   **Friday:** Lower
- **Push/Pull/Legs (PPL)** (4-6x per week): This split can be done either 3, 4, or 6 days per week. Rotate through Push, Pull, and Legs in that order.

  - o   **3x per week:** Push, Pull, Legs, rest, repeat.
  - o   **4x per week:** Push, Pull, Legs, rest, and pick up where you left off.
  - o   **6x per week:** Push, Pull, Legs, repeat cycle continuously.
- **Calisthenics Routine** (3-4x per week): Alternate **Workout A** and **Workout B**:

  - o   **Monday:** Workout A
  - o   **Wednesday:** Workout B
  - o   **Friday:** Workout A
  - o   **Next week:** Start with Workout B

Rest Periods: Timing for Maximum Efficiency

Rest periods are essential for recovery between sets, but the length of your rest will vary depending on the goal of your workout:

1. **For Fat Loss & Cardiovascular Fitness**:
   Shorter rest periods (30-60 seconds) keep your heart rate elevated and burn more calories. Ideal for circuits, supersets, and full-body routines.

2. **For Strength Building**:
   Longer rest periods (2-3 minutes) allow you to recover fully between heavy lifts. Best for compound movements like squats and deadlifts in the Upper/Lower or PPL splits.

3. **For Muscle Hypertrophy**:
   Moderate rest periods (60-90 seconds) balance muscle fatigue and volume. This is effective for routines focused on building muscle mass while maintaining a good tempo.

Post-Workout Stretching: Cooling Down for Recovery

Stretching after your workout helps reduce muscle stiffness, improve flexibility, and promote faster recovery. Focus on static stretches to lengthen the muscles that were just worked.

1. **Upper Body Stretches**:

   - **Chest Stretch**: Hold arms out wide and stretch across a door frame.
   - **Triceps Stretch**: Reach one arm overhead, bending the elbow, and use the opposite hand to push the elbow down gently.
   - **Shoulder Stretch**: Bring one arm across your chest and pull gently with the other arm.

2. **Lower Body Stretches**:

   - **Hamstring Stretch**: Sit with legs extended, reach toward your toes, and hold.
   - **Quad Stretch**: Stand on one leg, pulling the opposite leg's heel toward your glutes.
   - **Hip Flexor Stretch**: Kneel on one knee, push your hips forward to stretch the front of your hip.

3. **Core Stretch**:

   - **Cobra Stretch**: Lie face down, then push your chest up with your hands, arching your back to stretch the abs.

Duration: Hold each stretch for 20-30 seconds, and repeat 2-3 times per muscle group.

Recovery & Rest Days: The Importance of Recovery

While your workout is important, so is rest. Your muscles grow and repair during recovery, not just during the workout.

- **Rest Days**: For splits that work muscle groups intensively (like Full Body or PPL), plan rest days or active recovery days (light walking or yoga) to give your muscles time to heal.
- **Sleep**: Aim for 7-9 hours of quality sleep every night, as it's crucial for recovery and overall health.
- **Nutrition**: Ensure you're eating enough protein and other nutrients to support muscle recovery and fat loss.

Full-Body vs. Upper/Lower vs. Push/Pull/Legs vs. Calisthenics: Which Is Best for Fat Loss?

When it comes to fat loss, the best routine is the one that suits your lifestyle, goals, and workout preferences. Each of these training splits has unique advantages that can contribute to burning fat and improving fitness, but the choice ultimately depends on your available time, fitness level, and how much you enjoy the process.

Full-Body Workouts: Efficiency for Busy Schedules

Best for: Beginners, busy individuals, and those looking for quick, effective sessions.

Advantages:

- Engages multiple muscle groups in one session, burning more calories overall.
- You can work out 2-3 times a week and still see results, making it ideal for people with limited time.
- Higher frequency of full-body stimulation promotes more frequent fat loss.

Drawbacks:

- Limited volume for each muscle group compared to splits.
- Fatigue might set in toward the end, affecting performance on later exercises.

Upper/Lower Split: Balanced Focus and Moderate Time Commitment

Best for: Intermediate lifters who want to focus more on specific muscle groups while still keeping workouts efficient.
Advantages:

- Allows for more recovery time between sessions targeting the same muscle group.
- With 4 sessions per week, you can balance intensity and recovery, ensuring progress without burning out.
- Promotes muscle growth while maintaining fat loss with the right cardio and nutrition plan.

Drawbacks:

- Requires more gym days per week compared to full-body routines.
- May not burn as many calories in a single session compared to full-body workouts.

Push/Pull/Legs (PPL): Muscle Group Focus with More Frequency

Best for: Advanced lifters and those who can dedicate 4-6 days per week to the gym.
Advantages:

- Provides enough volume per muscle group to build muscle, which supports fat loss by increasing metabolism.
- Frequent training helps improve muscle endurance and cardiovascular conditioning.
- Easily tailored to fat loss goals by adding cardio or reducing rest times.

Drawbacks:

- Requires a higher time commitment and more frequent gym visits.
- If recovery is insufficient, fatigue can build up over the week, affecting performance.

Calisthenics: Functional Strength and Fat Loss with Minimal Equipment

Best for: People who prefer bodyweight exercises, want functional strength, or have minimal equipment.

Advantages:

- Can be done anywhere, making it highly convenient.
- Exercises like push-ups, pull-ups, and bodyweight squats burn calories while building lean muscle.
- Encourages movement patterns that engage core muscles and improve overall mobility and fitness.

Drawbacks:

- Limited potential for progressive overload compared to weight training.
- May require modifications or equipment (like resistance bands or weighted vests) to maintain progression over time.

Which One Should You Choose?

- **For Busy Schedules:** Go with Full-Body or Calisthenics routines for efficiency and flexibility.
- **For Moderate Commitment:** Upper/Lower splits offer a balanced approach between strength and fat loss.
- **For Maximum Focus and Volume:** PPL provides more volume and attention to each muscle group, ideal if you can commit to 4-6 gym days per week.

Ultimately, the best workout routine for fat loss is the one you can stay consistent with and enjoy over time.

Incorporating Cardio for Fat Loss

Cardio plays an essential role in boosting fat loss alongside strength training. While strength training focuses on building muscle and elevating metabolism, cardio helps increase calorie burn and enhance cardiovascular health. But which type of cardio is best for fat loss? Let's break it down.

Types of Cardio: HIIT vs. Steady-State Cardio

Both High-Intensity Interval Training (HIIT) and steady-state cardio are effective tools for fat loss, but they offer different benefits depending on your goals, time availability, and fitness level.

1. High-Intensity Interval Training (HIIT)

Definition: Alternates between intense bursts of exercise and short periods of rest or lower-intensity movements.

- **Duration:** Typically 20-30 minutes.
- **Intensity:** Maximum effort during work intervals (e.g., sprinting, cycling, or burpees) followed by lower intensity for recovery (e.g., walking or light jogging).

Benefits:

- **Time-Efficient:** HIIT sessions are short but effective, perfect for those with a tight schedule.
- **Afterburn Effect (EPOC):** HIIT increases your metabolism even after the workout, continuing to burn calories for hours post-exercise.
- **Increased Fat Burn:** Studies show that HIIT can lead to more significant fat loss compared to steady-state cardio in less time.

2. Steady-State Cardio

Definition: Maintaining a consistent, moderate intensity throughout the workout, such as jogging, brisk walking, or cycling at a steady pace.

- **Duration:** 30-60 minutes or more.
- **Intensity:** Moderate, about 50-70% of your max heart rate, meaning you can sustain the pace but still feel challenged.

Benefits:

- **Great for Beginners:** Easy to perform and maintain for longer durations.
- **Improves Endurance:** Builds aerobic capacity and helps improve overall cardiovascular health.
- **Low Impact:** Activities like walking or cycling are gentler on the joints compared to high-impact exercises.

When to Do Cardio: Before or After Strength Training?

The timing of cardio can influence how well your body performs during workouts and how efficiently you burn fat.

- **Cardio Before Strength Training:**
  Doing cardio before lifting weights might be useful if your primary goal is to improve cardiovascular fitness. However, this approach can fatigue your muscles and limit strength gains, which could hinder your ability to lift heavier or perform strength exercises effectively.

- **Cardio After Strength Training:**
  For fat loss, it's generally better to perform cardio after your strength workout. This ensures that you can put your full energy into lifting, helping to build muscle, which in turn boosts metabolism. Following up with cardio can increase calorie burn and assist with fat loss without compromising muscle gains.

HIIT Workouts for Fat Loss

Sample HIIT Routine 1: (20-30 minutes)

- Sprint (30 seconds)
- Rest (90 seconds)
- Repeat 8-10 times

Sample HIIT Routine 2:

- Jump Squats (30 seconds)
- Rest (15 seconds)
- Burpees (30 seconds)
- Rest (15 seconds)
- Mountain Climbers (30 seconds)
- Rest (15 seconds)
- Repeat for 4-5 rounds

Why HIIT Works for Fat Loss:

- **Afterburn Effect (EPOC):** HIIT is great for creating the "afterburn effect," scientifically known as Excess Post-Exercise Oxygen Consumption (EPOC). This means you'll continue to burn calories long after the workout is over, boosting fat loss while at rest.
- **Maximized Calorie Burn in Less Time:** You can achieve similar or even greater fat loss results in less time compared to longer steady-state sessions.

Steady-State Cardio Options

1. Walking

One of the most underrated forms of cardio, walking can be done anywhere and is easy to incorporate into your daily routine.

- **Duration:** 30-60 minutes
- **Intensity:** Brisk walking at 50-60% of your max heart rate.

2. Cycling

Cycling is a low-impact cardio option that strengthens your legs while improving cardiovascular fitness.

- **Duration:** 30-45 minutes
- **Intensity:** Maintain a steady pace or incorporate intervals to challenge yourself.

3. Rowing

Rowing engages your entire body, making it a great steady-state option for fat loss.

- **Duration:** 30 minutes
- **Intensity:** Moderate pace, focus on consistent strokes.

The Best Time for Steady-State Cardio: For optimal fat-burning results, steady-state cardio is often recommended in a fasted state (such as in the morning before breakfast). While research on fasted cardio's effectiveness is mixed, many people find it helps boost fat loss when combined with a proper nutrition plan.

Key Takeaways:

- **HIIT for Time Efficiency:** Perfect for busy schedules and those looking to maximize fat loss in less time.
- **Steady-State for Endurance:** Great for beginners, low-impact recovery sessions, and improving overall fitness.
- **Cardio Timing:** Perform cardio after strength training for maximum fat loss benefits without compromising muscle gains.

Both HIIT and steady-state cardio have their place in a fat loss plan, and alternating between the two can keep your workouts varied and exciting.

Progression and Tracking

Tracking Your Workouts

If you're serious about losing fat and building strength, tracking your workouts is non-negotiable. Whether it's strength training or cardio, having a system to record your progress keeps you accountable and helps you spot trends over time. There are several ways to track your workouts:

- **Apps**: With a plethora of fitness apps available on the App Store and Google Play Store, you can easily log every set, rep, and weight lifted. Some apps even let you track your cardio, offering insights on your progress, intensity, and overall performance. Many apps provide visual charts and graphs so you can see your progression at a glance.

- **Old School**: If you prefer a more hands-on approach, go old school with a pen and notebook. Keeping a physical journal of your workouts is a time-tested method. You can make notes about how you felt during a session, jot down personal bests, and stay organized without distractions from your phone.

- **Modernized Old School**: For those who want something a bit more convenient but still simple, using the Notes app on your phone works just as well. You can create a weekly log with exercises, sets, reps, and weights, adding any additional comments you feel are helpful (like how you felt during a workout or areas you want to improve).

When it comes to measuring fat loss, the scale might not always tell the full story. Muscle weighs more than fat, so as you get leaner and stronger, the scale might stay the same or even go up. That's why it's important to use multiple tools to track your fat loss:

- **The Mirror**: Sometimes, the best way to track your progress is with your own eyes. Take progress photos every couple of weeks in the same lighting and pose to notice subtle changes in your physique.

- **Body Measurements**: Measure key areas of your body—waist, hips, chest, arms, legs—every couple of weeks. Inches lost around your waist or hips might not show up on the scale, but these changes are a clear sign you're losing fat.

- **Body Fat Percentage**: If possible, use tools like body fat calipers or body fat scales to track your percentage of body fat. Even if the scale number stays the same, a drop in body fat means you're losing fat and gaining muscle—a win-win situation.

- **Scale Caution**: The scale can lie, especially when you're building muscle while losing fat. Don't obsess over it. Instead, focus on how your clothes fit, how you look in the mirror, and how your strength levels are improving.

Progression Tips

Progression is the key to fat loss and muscle building. As your body adapts to your current routine, you'll need to push it further to continue seeing results. This concept, called **progressive overload**, is all about gradually increasing the demands on your muscles and cardiovascular system to keep driving progress.

Increasing Weights or Reps

The simplest form of progression is to gradually increase the weights you're lifting. If you've been lifting the same weight for the same number of reps for 2-3 workouts, it's time to either increase the weight or try to get an extra rep or two. This ensures you're constantly challenging your muscles and pushing them to grow.

Cardio Intensity

When it comes to cardio, progression could mean increasing the intensity of your sessions. For example, if you're doing High-Intensity Interval Training (HIIT), you can shorten the rest periods or increase the speed during the work intervals. If you're doing steady-state cardio like running or cycling, increase the speed, incline, or resistance over time to boost fat loss.

Varying Exercises and Workout Plans

To avoid plateaus, it's important to adjust your exercises when you notice signs that your body
has adapted to the current routine. While 6-8 weeks is a general recommendation, the key is to
listen to your body. If you notice that the weight you're lifting isn't increasing, your reps are
going down, or you're not feeling the same challenge from your workouts, it might be time to
switch things up.

This could be as simple as:

- **Changing from Barbell to Dumbbell Variations**: Swapping between barbells and
  dumbbells can engage stabilizing muscles differently and provide a new stimulus for
  growth.
- **Alternative Exercises**: You can switch out certain exercises for alternatives that target
  the same muscle group. For example, replace barbell squats with front squats, or
  dumbbell bench press with a cable press.
- **Change Rep Schemes**: Adjusting the number of reps and sets can also spark new
  progress. If you've been working in the 6-8 rep range for a while, try increasing to 10-12
  reps or even 15 reps to increase endurance and challenge your muscles differently.

On a more personal note, I like to keep things fresh by cycling between 2-3 different workout
plans. Each plan is designed to target a specific goal—whether it's strength, hypertrophy, or fat
loss. When I feel like I'm getting bored or hitting a plateau, I switch things up. For instance:

- **For Strength**: I focus on heavier weights, fewer reps, and more rest between sets.
- **For Hypertrophy**: I switch to moderate weights with higher reps and shorter rest
  times to push muscle growth.
- **For Weight Loss**: I shift to higher volume or circuit-style training with added cardio.

By actively rotating between these workout plans, you can continue to challenge your body,
avoid stagnation, and stay motivated to achieve your goals. It's not just about physical
adaptation, but **mental fatigue** too—sometimes you need that variety to stay engaged and
excited about your workouts.

Recovery and Adaptation

The importance of recovery can't be overstated. It's during the recovery process that your
muscles repair and grow stronger. If you're not allowing enough recovery time, you're not only
hindering fat loss and muscle growth, but you also risk injury.

Resting Between Workouts

Each muscle group needs 48-72 hours to recover fully before you target it again. Full-body routines should be spaced out with at least one day of rest between sessions, while split routines (like Upper/Lower or PPL) should have rest days built into the schedule to avoid overworking the same muscles. Personally, I rarely plan deload weeks because life tends to do it for me. Whether it's getting sick, having a ton of work piled up, or dealing with family matters, these unplanned breaks can force me to rest. While it may not always come at the most convenient time, these moments are a reminder that rest is essential, even when it's not scheduled.

However, if you're consistently hitting your workouts hard, incorporating **deload weeks—** periods where you intentionally reduce workout intensity or volume—can be beneficial. These weeks allow your body to recover, helping to prevent overtraining and injury while preparing you to come back stronger for your next round of workouts.

Stretching and Mobility

Stretching after your workouts can improve flexibility and help prevent injury. It also aids in muscle recovery by increasing blood flow to the muscles. Incorporating mobility work, such as **dynamic stretching** before workouts and **static stretching** afterward, helps your body stay limber and reduces muscle soreness.

Examples of Dynamic Stretches (Pre-Workout):

- **Leg Swings:** Helps to open up the hips and improve range of motion for lower-body exercises like squats.
- **Arm Circles:** A great way to loosen up your shoulders before pressing movements.
- **Hip Circles:** Prepares your hips for any heavy lifting or leg work.

Examples of Static Stretches (Post-Workout):

- **Hamstring Stretch:** Targets the hamstrings, especially after exercises like deadlifts or leg presses.
- **Chest Stretch:** Opens up the chest muscles after upper-body pressing workouts.
- **Child's Pose:** A relaxing way to stretch your back and shoulders after a workout.

Incorporating **dead hangs** into your routine can also be beneficial. A dead hang involves hanging from a pull-up bar with your arms fully extended, allowing your body to decompress and relieve tension in the spine. To perform a dead hang:

1. Grip the bar with both hands, palms facing away from you, and allow your body to hang straight down.
2. Keep your shoulders engaged and avoid letting them rise toward your ears.
3. Hold the position for 20-30 seconds, focusing on deep breathing and relaxation.

This exercise not only aids in spinal decompression but also helps improve grip strength and shoulder stability.

Active Recovery

On your rest days, consider incorporating **active recovery** methods such as light cardio, stretching, or foam rolling. These activities help keep your muscles loose and promote blood flow without putting undue stress on your body. Active recovery is a great way to facilitate recovery while staying engaged in movement.

In addition to traditional forms of active recovery, everyday activities can also contribute to keeping your body moving. Tasks such as cleaning up after children, vacuuming the house, or mowing the lawn can serve as effective ways to stay active.

However, it's essential to remember that it's still a rest day. Enjoy your progress and allow your body the time it needs to recover fully. Balancing movement with relaxation will help you come back stronger for your next workout.

Sleep and Nutrition

Rest is an integral part of your fitness journey. Ensure you're prioritizing quality sleep and proper nutrition to support muscle repair and fat loss. Without adequate rest and fuel, your body won't perform at its best, and your results will suffer.

Focus on protein intake to facilitate muscle recovery. Post-workout meals are crucial for replenishing energy, so include a balance of carbohydrates and protein to restore glycogen levels and promote muscle repair. Additionally, staying hydrated throughout the day is essential for overall performance and recovery.

Common Mistakes to Avoid

1. Overtraining

Introduction to Overtraining

Overtraining occurs when an individual exceeds their body's ability to recover from strenuous exercise, leading to physical and mental fatigue. While it's natural to push yourself in your fitness journey, doing so excessively without allowing adequate rest can have detrimental effects.

Definition of Overtraining

Overtraining is characterized by a state of physical and psychological exhaustion caused by excessive training without sufficient recovery. When the body is consistently subjected to high levels of stress, it can't repair itself properly, leading to a range of negative outcomes.

Symptoms of Overtraining

Recognizing the signs of overtraining is crucial for anyone looking to achieve their fitness goals. Common symptoms include:

- **Fatigue:** A pervasive sense of tiredness that doesn't improve with rest.
- **Decreased Performance:** A noticeable drop in strength, endurance, and overall workout performance, which can be frustrating and disheartening.
- **Irritability:** Heightened mood swings and irritability, often due to hormonal imbalances that can result from chronic stress.
- **Insomnia:** Difficulty falling or staying asleep, leading to a cycle of fatigue that further hampers recovery.
- **Increased Injuries:** An uptick in injuries or persistent soreness, indicating that the body is not recovering properly.

Impact on Weight Loss and Overall Progress

Overtraining can significantly hinder weight loss efforts and overall fitness progress. When the body is in a state of fatigue, it becomes less efficient at burning calories and building muscle. Hormonal imbalances can lead to increased cortisol levels, a stress hormone that can promote fat storage, especially around the abdomen.

Moreover, the psychological toll of overtraining can lead to a decrease in motivation and consistency. Individuals may feel discouraged by their performance dips, potentially leading them to abandon their fitness routines altogether. In this way, the cycle of overtraining can create setbacks that are counterproductive to the goals of weight loss and improved fitness.

To prevent overtraining, it's essential to listen to your body, incorporate rest days into your routine, and maintain a balanced approach to exercise that prioritizes both intensity and recovery.

1. Why More Isn't Always Better

In the pursuit of fitness goals, a common misconception prevails: the belief that spending more hours in the gym guarantees better results. Many individuals equate longer workout sessions with greater dedication and progress, leading them to adopt grueling training schedules that can ultimately backfire.

The Misconception of Workout Duration

While it's true that consistency and effort are crucial for success, simply adding more hours to your training doesn't automatically translate to improved performance or results. In fact, overemphasis on duration can lead to diminishing returns. Research shows that beyond a certain point, additional workout time can lead to fatigue and decreased effectiveness, resulting in poor form and increased risk of injury.

Quality Over Quantity

Instead of focusing solely on the number of hours spent exercising, it's vital to prioritize the quality of workouts. This means engaging in targeted, well-structured training sessions that challenge the body while allowing for proper recovery.

The Importance of Rest and Recovery

Rest and recovery are essential components of an effective fitness regimen. They provide the body with the necessary time to repair itself and adapt to the stresses of exercise. Skipping rest days or minimizing recovery can lead to a host of negative outcomes, including burnout, overtraining, and injuries.

1. **Muscle Repair and Growth:**

   o   During exercise, particularly resistance training, tiny tears occur in muscle fibers. Rest days are when the body repairs these fibers, leading to muscle growth and strength gains. This recovery period is essential for progress; without it, muscles remain in a constant state of stress, leading to stagnation or decline.

2. **Hormonal Balance:**

   o   Adequate recovery helps maintain hormonal balance. Overtraining can elevate cortisol levels, which is linked to stress and can impede muscle growth while promoting fat storage. Prioritizing recovery helps keep hormones in check, allowing for optimal performance and results.

3. **Mental Health:**

   o   Beyond physical benefits, recovery plays a vital role in mental well-being. Overtraining can lead to mental fatigue and a lack of motivation, making it harder to maintain a consistent workout routine. Incorporating rest days allows for mental rejuvenation, keeping the enthusiasm for training alive.

Conclusion: Time to Recover, Time to Grow

In summary, while the hustle and grind mentality can be motivating, it's crucial to remember that more isn't always better when it comes to workouts. Embracing a balanced approach that includes adequate rest and recovery will ultimately lead to better results, improved performance, and a sustainable fitness journey. By prioritizing recovery, you set yourself up for success, ensuring that your muscles have the time they need to repair and grow stronger.

2. How to Avoid Burnout

Preventing burnout is crucial for maintaining a sustainable and effective fitness regimen. Here are three key strategies to help you stay energized and motivated throughout your journey.

1. Listening to Your Body

One of the most important aspects of avoiding burnout is learning to listen to your body. Your body is a highly adaptive system that provides signals when it needs attention. Recognizing these signs can help you prevent overtraining and its associated effects.

- **Pay Attention to Signs of Fatigue:**
    - Fatigue isn't just about feeling tired; it can manifest as decreased motivation, persistent soreness, or a lack of enthusiasm for workouts. If you notice these signs, it may be time to scale back and allow for recovery.
- **Recognize Soreness vs. Pain:**
    - Understanding the difference between general muscle soreness (which is normal) and acute pain (which could indicate injury) is vital. If you experience sharp or persistent pain, it's essential to rest and consult a professional if needed.
- **Keep a Training Journal:**
    - Maintaining a log of your workouts, how you feel during and after sessions, and any signs of fatigue can help you identify patterns. This can guide your training decisions and highlight when to push harder or take a step back.

2. Implementing Rest Days

Rest days are not a sign of weakness; rather, they are a fundamental component of a successful training plan. Scheduling regular rest days allows your body to recover, adapt, and ultimately improve.

- **Balanced Routine:**
    - Aim for a balanced workout routine that includes both training days and rest days. For example, consider a schedule that alternates between intense workout days and lighter or rest days. A common approach is training hard for 3-5 days, followed by at least 1-2 days of rest or active recovery.

- **Active Recovery:**

  - o   On rest days, consider engaging in light activities like walking, stretching, or yoga. This keeps the body moving without the strain of high-intensity workouts and promotes blood flow to aid recovery.

3. Cross-Training

Cross-training involves incorporating a variety of workout types into your routine, which can help prevent burnout and keep things fresh and exciting.

- **Benefits of Varying Workouts:**

  - o   Engaging in different types of exercises—such as cycling, swimming, yoga, or strength training—helps work various muscle groups, reduces the risk of overuse injuries, and can enhance overall fitness levels.

- **Mental Engagement:**

  - o   Trying new activities can boost motivation and enjoyment. If you find yourself getting bored with your usual routine, mixing in different workouts can reignite your passion for fitness.

- **Example Cross-Training Activities:**

  - o   Consider adding activities like hiking, dance classes, or team sports to your schedule. Not only does this introduce variety, but it also allows you to socialize and build community while staying active.

Conclusion

By listening to your body, implementing regular rest days, and incorporating cross-training into your routine, you can significantly reduce the risk of burnout. These strategies foster a balanced approach to fitness, allowing for consistent progress while promoting overall well-being. Remember, recovery is just as important as the work you put in; prioritize it to achieve sustainable success on your fitness journey.

Ignoring Strength Training

The Role of Strength Training in Fat Loss

Strength training plays a crucial role in any effective fat loss program. It involves exercises that challenge your muscles against resistance, leading to numerous benefits.

- **Building Muscle Increases Metabolism:**

  - One of the primary advantages of strength training is its ability to build lean muscle mass. Unlike fat, muscle tissue requires more energy to maintain, which means that the more muscle you have, the higher your resting metabolic rate. This increased metabolism helps your body burn more calories even at rest, making it easier to achieve and maintain fat loss.

- **Improving Body Composition:**

  - When it comes to fat loss, body composition is just as important as the number on the scale. Strength training helps reduce body fat while preserving muscle mass, resulting in a more toned and defined physique. In contrast, relying solely on cardio for weight loss often leads to muscle loss, which can negatively impact metabolism and overall health.

1. The Misconception: Cardio vs. Strength Training

A common belief in the fitness community is that cardio is the only way to lose weight effectively. Many people gravitate towards running, cycling, or other forms of cardiovascular exercise, believing that these activities alone will deliver the best results.

- **Evidence Against the Myth:**

  - While cardio is beneficial for cardiovascular health and can aid in burning calories, research indicates that strength training can be equally, if not more, effective for fat loss. Studies show that individuals who incorporate strength training into their routine tend to lose more fat and maintain muscle mass compared to those who rely solely on cardio.

- **The Synergy of Both:**

  o The most effective approach to fat loss combines both strength training and cardio. Each serves a unique purpose, and together they can create a balanced fitness regimen that enhances overall health and weight loss results.

2. Incorporating Strength Training into Your Routine

Incorporating strength training into your routine is essential for maximizing fat loss and improving overall fitness. Here are some effective exercises to consider:

- **Squats:** A foundational lower-body exercise that targets the quads, hamstrings, and glutes.
- **Deadlifts:** A full-body exercise that primarily works the posterior chain, including the back, glutes, and hamstrings.
- **Push-Ups:** A bodyweight exercise that strengthens the chest, shoulders, and triceps while engaging the core.
- **Lunges:** A versatile exercise that targets the legs and improves balance and coordination.
- **Plank:** An excellent core-strengthening exercise that also engages the shoulders and glutes.

Conclusion

Ignoring strength training can be a significant mistake in the journey toward fat loss and improved health. By understanding its vital role, addressing common misconceptions, and actively incorporating strength training into your routine, you can enhance your body composition and achieve sustainable weight loss. Embrace the challenge of strength training to maximize your results!

3. Skipping Progressive Overload

Understanding Progressive Overload

Progressive overload is a fundamental principle in strength training and an essential component of any successful fat loss program. It involves gradually increasing the intensity of your workouts over time to continuously challenge your muscles.

- **Definition and Importance:**
  - Progressive overload means systematically increasing the amount of stress placed on your body during exercise. This can be achieved through various means, such as lifting heavier weights, increasing the number of repetitions or sets, or reducing rest times between sets. The importance of this principle lies in its ability to stimulate muscle growth and adaptation, leading to improved strength, endurance, and overall fitness.
- **Continuous Progress:**
  - Gradually increasing the intensity of your workouts ensures that your body doesn't adapt too quickly. When you provide a consistent challenge, your muscles are forced to grow stronger and more resilient, which ultimately contributes to fat loss and enhanced performance.

How Staying in Your Comfort Zone Slows Progress

While it can be tempting to stick with familiar weights and routines, doing so can significantly hinder your progress.

- **The Dangers of Stagnation:**
  - Continuing to perform the same exercises with the same weights can lead to plateaus, where your progress stalls, and you may not see any further improvements in strength or body composition. This stagnation can be frustrating and demotivating, making it easy to lose sight of your fitness goals.
- **Examples of Plateauing:**
  - For instance, if you've been performing bicep curls with the same weight for several weeks, your muscles will eventually adapt to that load. Without a challenge, there's no stimulus for growth, and you may find it difficult to increase your strength or muscle size. The body requires progressive challenges

to keep evolving, and without them, you risk becoming complacent in your training.

Tips for Implementing Progressive Overload

Incorporating progressive overload into your fitness routine is crucial for continued progress. Here are some effective strategies to help you implement this principle:

- **Increase Weights:**

    o   As you become stronger, gradually increase the weights you use in your workouts. Aim for small increments (e.g., 2.5 to 5 pounds) to ensure you can maintain proper form while challenging your muscles.

- **Vary Repetitions and Sets:**

    o   Adjust the number of repetitions and sets in your workouts. For instance, if you typically perform three sets of 10 reps, try increasing to three sets of 12 or adding an additional set. This variation keeps your workouts challenging and stimulates muscle growth.

- **Modify Exercise Variations:**

    o   Explore different variations of exercises to target the same muscle groups from various angles. For example, if you usually do standard squats, try adding sumo squats, front squats, or split squats. This diversity not only keeps workouts interesting but also helps to prevent plateaus.

Conclusion

Avoiding the mistake of skipping progressive overload is vital for anyone serious about their fitness journey. By understanding its importance and implementing strategies to ensure continuous challenge, you can maximize your strength training results and enhance your fat loss efforts. Remember to maintain a balance between challenge and recovery, combining rest, strength training, and progressive overload for optimal results.

Chapter 3 Conclusion: You've Started—Keep It Going

As we wrap up this chapter on effective workout plans, understand the multifaceted approach needed for building muscle, improving health, and maximizing fat loss. By implementing the strategies and insights shared here, you can craft a personalized fitness routine that aligns with your goals.

Key Takeaways:

- **Balanced Approach:** Optimal results require a blend of strength training and cardiovascular exercise. Both are vital for enhancing metabolic function and promoting fat loss.

- **The Importance of Strength Training:** Strength training is key for building muscle, increasing your resting metabolic rate, and supporting long-term fat loss. Focus on compound movements and apply progressive overload to continuously challenge your body.

- **Incorporating Cardio:** Whether you choose High-Intensity Interval Training (HIIT) or steady-state cardio, integrating cardiovascular workouts effectively accelerates fat loss and boosts overall fitness.

- **Tracking Progress:** Keep a detailed log of your workouts and monitor progress using various metrics beyond the scale. Adjust your routines based on your advancements to prevent plateaus and sustain motivation.

- **Avoiding Common Pitfalls:** Be aware of common mistakes like overtraining, neglecting strength training, and failing to implement progressive overload. Listen to your body; it's essential for long-term success.

Reaching this point in your fitness journey is already a significant achievement. Your commitment to learning and improving is what truly matters. Consistency is crucial, but ensure you create a routine that feels sustainable and enjoyable.

Embrace the process—each workout, healthy choice, and small step forward contributes to your progress. Be patient and stay focused on your goals, recognizing that real transformation takes time and effort.

With the right mindset and a solid workout plan, you have everything you need to achieve lasting results. Keep pushing forward, trust in your ability, and take action today. Your journey is just beginning, and the best is yet to come!

Chapter 4: Recovery: The Missing Piece

I. Introduction to Recovery

1. Why Recovery is Key to Fat Loss and Muscle Growth

Understanding the Role of Recovery in Progress
Recovery isn't just about taking a day off from the gym. It's the period during which your body heals and adapts to the stress of exercise. Every time you engage in intense workouts—whether it's lifting weights, running, or doing HIIT—you're causing microscopic damage to muscle fibers. This is normal and part of the process, but it's the **repair of these fibers during rest** that makes them stronger and leaner.

The Link Between Recovery and Fat Loss
In terms of fat loss, recovery plays a pivotal role because a body under constant stress can struggle to burn fat effectively. Overtraining raises cortisol levels, a stress hormone linked to fat retention, particularly around the abdomen. When you allow your body to recover, cortisol levels normalize, and the metabolic processes involved in burning fat work more efficiently. Also, **muscles burn more calories at rest**, so the more lean muscle you build through proper recovery, the higher your overall calorie burn will be—even when you're not exercising.

2. The Overlooked Importance of Rest

Rest Days Are Not Lazy Days
Many people equate taking a rest day with slacking off, but this couldn't be further from the truth. Rest days are when your muscles actually grow stronger. Without them, your body doesn't have enough time to repair itself, leading to **fatigue, decreased performance**, and **mental burnout**. Over time, this can cause you to feel unmotivated, frustrated by a lack of progress, or worse, injured.

The Science of Overtraining and Its Impact on Results
When you train without adequate recovery, you risk entering a state of **overtraining syndrome**. This condition can lead to:

- **Decreased immune function**, making you more susceptible to illnesses.

- **Hormonal imbalances**, including elevated cortisol and reduced testosterone, both of which negatively impact fat loss and muscle gain.
- **Chronic fatigue** and **joint pain**, which reduce the effectiveness of future workouts and increase injury risks.

The Importance of Sleep in Recovery

A key aspect of recovery is sleep, which is when your body undergoes the most profound repair and regeneration. During sleep, the release of **growth hormone** peaks, which is essential for muscle recovery and fat loss. Lack of sleep has been shown to slow muscle repair, hinder fat loss, and increase cravings for unhealthy foods due to the impact on hunger-regulating hormones like **ghrelin** and **leptin**.

3. Practical Recovery Strategies

Incorporating Active Recovery

Active recovery, such as **light walking**, **stretching**, or **yoga**, can be a great way to promote blood flow to sore muscles without overloading them. These low-intensity activities enhance recovery without stressing your body further, helping to reduce muscle soreness (DOMS) and keeping you moving even on rest days.

Scheduling Rest and Recovery Days

Proper recovery is about balancing intense workout days with rest. A general rule of thumb is to schedule at least **1-2 full rest days per week**, especially when engaging in high-intensity strength training or cardio. Alternatively, using a split routine (e.g., alternating upper-body and lower-body workouts) can allow specific muscle groups to recover while others are being worked, providing partial recovery even while staying active.

The Science of Recovery

1. Muscle Repair and Growth

Breaking Down to Build Back Stronger

Every time you lift weights or engage in intense physical activity, you create **microtears** in your muscle fibers. These tiny tears are a natural part of muscle growth, but they require proper recovery for repair. During the recovery phase, your body works to **repair these tears** by fusing muscle fibers together, making them stronger and larger. This process is called **muscle hypertrophy**—the growth of muscle mass.

The Anabolic Window: Myth vs. Reality

After your workout, your body enters a state known as the **anabolic phase**, where it begins the process of muscle repair and growth. Many people have heard of the "anabolic window"—the idea that you need to consume **protein and carbohydrates** within a strict 30-minute window post-workout to avoid losing gains.

This is total BS.

While nutrient timing **does** matter, the idea that you need to chug a protein shake immediately after your workout or risk losing muscle is a **myth**. Yes, consuming protein and carbohydrates post-workout helps supply your muscles with the building blocks they need for repair (amino acids from protein and glycogen replenishment from carbs), but the so-called "anabolic window" is **much larger** than 30 minutes. Studies have shown that **as long as you get sufficient protein within a few hours after your workout**, you'll still support muscle repair and growth. In fact, the total amount of protein you consume throughout the day is far more important than rushing to hit an arbitrary post-workout window.

Delayed-Onset Muscle Soreness (DOMS)

You've probably experienced DOMS, the soreness that sets in 24 to 48 hours after an intense workout. This soreness is a sign of muscle damage, but it's also an indicator that your muscles are adapting to the workload. While DOMS is a natural part of the recovery process, excessive soreness may signal overtraining or poor recovery habits, which can hinder progress. Balancing intensity with proper recovery is essential to avoid prolonged soreness that can interrupt your workout routine.

2. The Role of the Nervous System

Understanding Central Nervous System (CNS) Fatigue

Recovery isn't just about repairing muscles; it's also about giving your **nervous system** time to recuperate. The **central nervous system (CNS)** is responsible for sending signals from your brain to your muscles, allowing you to lift, push, and move with power and precision. After intense training, especially heavy lifting or high-intensity cardio, the CNS becomes fatigued. This is why you might feel mentally and physically drained after a hard workout, even if your muscles aren't particularly sore.

CNS Fatigue vs. Muscle Fatigue

While muscle fatigue is often more obvious (soreness, stiffness), CNS fatigue can be harder to detect. Symptoms include:

- **Lack of focus** or mental fog.
- **Reduced coordination** or reaction time.
- **Lowered motivation** to work out.

Recovery for the CNS

Unlike muscles, which benefit from targeted stretching or foam rolling, the nervous system recovers primarily through **rest**. This makes sleep and overall rest days critical components of your fitness routine. Without adequate recovery time, CNS fatigue can accumulate, leading to diminished performance and the potential for injury. Ensuring you're not constantly pushing your body to its limits without allowing your CNS to recover is vital for long-term progress.

3. Hormonal Balance

Cortisol: The Stress Hormone

Cortisol is often referred to as the **stress hormone** because it is released in response to physical and mental stress, including intense exercise. While cortisol is necessary for energy production and regulating metabolism, **chronically elevated cortisol levels** due to overtraining or insufficient recovery can have negative effects. These include:

- **Muscle breakdown** (catabolism), hindering muscle repair and growth.
- **Fat retention**, particularly around the midsection.
- Increased cravings for sugary or high-fat foods.

Adequate recovery—both physical and mental—helps lower cortisol levels, allowing your body to shift from a **catabolic**(breakdown) state to an **anabolic** (building) state, which is essential for muscle growth and fat loss.

Growth Hormone: The Recovery Accelerator

During deep sleep, the body releases **growth hormone (GH)**, which plays a crucial role in muscle recovery, fat metabolism, and overall tissue repair. GH promotes the synthesis of new proteins, which are necessary for repairing damaged muscle fibers. This hormone also aids in **fat burning**, making it a powerful tool for both muscle building and fat loss.

However, **poor sleep habits** or chronic stress can decrease the release of growth hormone, slowing down your body's ability to repair and recover. This is why sleep quality is just as important as sleep quantity—ensuring you get **deep, restful sleep** allows your body to maximize its growth hormone production.

Testosterone: The Muscle-Building Hormone

Testosterone is the primary hormone responsible for **muscle growth** in both men and women. It plays a significant role in increasing protein synthesis, which helps in building and repairing muscle tissue. Inadequate recovery, high stress levels, and lack of sleep can all reduce testosterone levels, leading to:

- Slower muscle growth.
- Decreased strength.
- Lower energy levels and motivation.

Maintaining balanced testosterone levels through proper recovery, stress management, and **healthy dietary choices**(including adequate fats and proteins) is essential for sustaining muscle growth and supporting overall fitness.

Practical Tips for Optimizing Hormonal Balance

- **Prioritize Sleep**: Aim for 7-9 hours of quality sleep each night to boost growth hormone production and lower cortisol.
- **Manage Stress**: Incorporate stress-relieving activities like meditation, yoga, or even light walks to keep cortisol levels in check.
- **Healthy Fats**: Include healthy fats in your diet (e.g., avocados, nuts, olive oil) to support testosterone production.

The Different Types of Recovery

1. Passive Recovery: Let Your Body Rest

Rest Days:

Planned rest days are non-negotiable for long-term progress. Your muscles don't grow during workouts—they grow during recovery. By incorporating scheduled rest days into your routine, you allow your body time to repair the micro-tears in muscle fibers caused by strength training. Rest days also help prevent overtraining, which can lead to burnout and increased risk of injury.

It's not just about resting your body; it's about resting your **mind** too. Rest days help reset your nervous system, giving it a break from the high-intensity signals it processes during workouts.

Sleep:

Quality sleep is often the most underestimated factor in recovery. During deep sleep (especially REM sleep), your body releases growth hormones that drive muscle repair and fat loss. Sleep also helps regulate cortisol levels—keeping stress in check. Research consistently shows that 7-9 hours of sleep per night is essential for optimal recovery and performance.

Lack of sleep not only affects physical recovery but can also throw off your metabolism and hunger hormones, making it harder to lose fat and build muscle.

Naps:

Napping can be a powerful tool in your recovery arsenal. Short naps of 20-30 minutes can help recharge your energy levels and improve cognitive function without causing sleep inertia, which can happen if you sleep too long. If you're feeling particularly drained after intense workouts or sleepless nights, a 90-minute nap allows you to complete a full sleep cycle, which can enhance muscle recovery and cognitive performance.

2. Active Recovery: Stay Moving Without Stressing the Body

Low-Intensity Activities:

Active recovery is a great way to keep moving while promoting recovery, as it increases blood flow to muscles without adding stress. Activities like walking, light stretching, or yoga can help reduce muscle soreness and stiffness. These low-intensity movements keep your joints and muscles active without overtaxing them, which aids in clearing metabolic waste like lactic acid and speeds up the recovery process.

Foam Rolling and Mobility Work:

Self-myofascial release techniques like foam rolling are vital for improving blood flow and releasing muscle tightness. Foam rolling works by breaking up scar tissue and adhesions in your muscles, which can build up after intense workouts. This not only enhances recovery but also helps improve your range of motion and prevent future injuries.

Mobility work goes hand in hand with foam rolling. Incorporating dynamic stretches, joint rotations, and functional movements enhances flexibility and keeps your body moving fluidly, which can drastically improve your workout performance and recovery. Think of this as maintaining the "software" of your body—keeping everything running smoothly for the long term.

Hot and Cold Baths:

Contrast baths, which involve alternating between hot and cold water immersion, can be beneficial for recovery by enhancing circulation, reducing muscle soreness, and promoting quicker elimination of metabolic waste. However, it's important to note that this method places additional stress on the body, as it forces your cardiovascular system to adapt to the sudden changes in temperature.

Individuals with heart conditions or those who are sensitive to temperature fluctuations should avoid this recovery method, as the stress on the body can exacerbate existing health issues. Always consult a healthcare professional before incorporating contrast baths into your routine if you have any underlying health concerns.

Stress Management and Recovery

1. **The Impact of Stress on Recovery and Fat Loss:** Chronic stress leads to elevated cortisol levels, a hormone that can negatively affect both fat loss and muscle recovery. High cortisol levels can cause the body to store more fat, particularly around the abdominal area, and make it harder for muscles to recover post-workout. Prolonged stress also compromises sleep quality, further hindering recovery and overall fitness progress.

2. **Mental Recovery:** Physical recovery isn't enough—mental recovery is just as crucial. Incorporate techniques like:

    o   **Meditation:** Regular practice can help reduce stress and lower cortisol levels, creating a more balanced environment for recovery.
    o   **Deep Breathing Exercises:** Simple breathing techniques can trigger relaxation, reduce stress, and enhance your body's ability to recover.
    o   **Mindfulness Practices:** Staying present and aware helps reduce anxiety, improve focus, and create a sense of calm, which aids in both mental and physical recovery.

3. **Balancing Training and Life Stress:** Training hard is important, but balancing it with life's other stressors is essential to avoid burnout. Some strategies include:

    o   **Listening to Your Body:** If you're mentally or physically exhausted from work, family, or other stress, scale back on training intensity rather than pushing through.

- o   **Flexible Scheduling**: Build your routine around your life commitments—train hard when you can, but don't stress about dialing it down when life gets hectic. Adaptability is key for long-term success.
- o   **Setting Boundaries**: Ensure your workout and recovery time remains a priority even amidst life's demands—protecting this time can actually enhance both your personal and professional life by keeping stress in check.

Stress is a Part of Life: It's easy for people to say, "Just stop stressing," but let's be real—that's not how life works. Stress is inevitable, and pretending you can just switch it off isn't realistic. I'm no psychologist, so I'm not here to tell you how to manage every aspect of it, but I can tell you what's worked for me during long periods of stress and stagnation.

What helped me the most was facing the causes head-on. Instead of letting the weight of ten different stressors crush me, I focused on tackling them one by one. By eliminating or dealing with the causes piece by piece, I gradually reduced the load. When I went from having 10 things stressing me out to just 1 or 2, everything became a lot more manageable.

This isn't a quick fix, but it's a real one. Sometimes, it's about taking the punch, rolling with it, and working through the tough stuff step by step.

Nutrition and Supplements for Optimal Recovery

Nutrition's Role in Recovery:

- **Protein:**
  Protein is the key building block for muscle repair, and the amount you need can vary depending on your goals, training intensity, and whether you're in a calorie deficit. Typically, the recommended intake is between 1.6 to 2.2 grams of protein per kilogram of body weight. However, when you're in a calorie deficit (cutting), it's beneficial to aim for the higher end of that range to preserve muscle mass and support recovery. Good sources include lean meats, fish, eggs, dairy, and plant-based options like beans and tofu. Distribute protein evenly throughout the day to optimize muscle repair and growth.

- **Carbohydrates:**
  Glycogen is the primary fuel your muscles use during workouts, and carbohydrates are essential for replenishing these stores. Post-workout, aim to consume fast-digesting

carbs (like fruits or white rice) within an hour of training to kickstart recovery. For overall daily intake, focus on complex carbs like oats, sweet potatoes, and whole grains to maintain energy levels and support muscle recovery over time.

- **Healthy Fats:**
  While carbohydrates and protein often get the spotlight in discussions of recovery, dietary fats play a critical role as well. Fats, particularly healthy fats from sources like avocados, nuts, seeds, olive oil, and fatty fish (rich in omega-3s), are essential for hormone production and regulation. Hormones such as testosterone and growth hormone, which are crucial for muscle growth and recovery, rely on adequate fat intake.

Hydration:

- Dehydration can significantly impact recovery, leading to muscle cramps, delayed recovery times, and a higher risk of injury. It's vital to drink water consistently throughout the day, especially before, during, and after workouts. For athletes training intensely or for long durations, incorporating a drink with added electrolytes can help maintain fluid balance and prevent issues like muscle cramps or dizziness.

Supplements:

- **Protein Powders:**
  Whey protein is quickly absorbed and ideal for consumption immediately post-workout, providing the muscles with the amino acids they need to jumpstart recovery. *Casein protein* digests slowly, making it beneficial before bed to support muscle repair throughout the night. Including both types in your nutrition plan can maximize recovery potential across the day.

- **BCAAs (Branched-Chain Amino Acids):**
  BCAAs, including leucine, isoleucine, and valine, are promoted for their role in stimulating muscle protein synthesis and reducing muscle soreness. While BCAAs may be helpful for people on low-protein diets, their benefits are less pronounced for those already consuming sufficient protein. They're most useful during prolonged exercise sessions where muscle breakdown could be more pronounced.

- **Creatine:**
  Creatine is one of the most studied and effective supplements for enhancing muscle recovery and performance. It works by replenishing ATP (your muscle's energy currency), which can help you push through tough workouts and recover faster. Regular creatine use has also been shown to improve strength gains and muscle mass, making it a solid option for anyone looking to improve both performance and recovery.

- **Electrolytes:**
  Sweating during workouts leads to the loss of important electrolytes, including sodium, potassium, and magnesium, which are critical for maintaining fluid balance and muscle function. Consider electrolyte drinks or supplements, especially after intense or prolonged exercise sessions, to aid in hydration and recovery. Coconut water or electrolyte-rich drinks can be natural and effective ways to restore these levels.

- **Sleep Supplements:**
  Adequate sleep is essential for recovery, but if you're struggling with sleep, supplements like *magnesium* can help relax muscles and nerves, promoting better sleep quality. *Melatonin*, a natural hormone, can aid in regulating your sleep cycle, especially if your sleep schedule is inconsistent. Improved sleep leads to better hormone regulation, muscle recovery, and overall performance.

Additional Supplements (if space allows):

- **Omega-3 Fatty Acids:**
  Omega-3s (found in fish oil or flaxseed supplements) can reduce muscle soreness and inflammation, enhancing recovery. They also support joint health, which can be especially beneficial if you're engaging in heavy lifting or intense cardio.

- **Vitamin D:**
  Low vitamin D levels have been linked to impaired muscle function and slower recovery. Supplementing vitamin D, especially during winter months or for those who spend a lot of time indoors, can aid muscle repair and overall immune function.

Wrapping Up Recovery: The Key to Long-Term Success

Recovery isn't just about resting; it's about giving your body the tools it needs to rebuild, recharge, and come back stronger. By prioritizing sleep, managing stress, and fueling your body with the right nutrients, you'll maximize your progress and reduce the risk of injury or burnout. Remember, recovery is not a luxury—it's a necessity for sustainable fat loss and muscle growth. Embrace it as a vital part of your routine, and you'll be setting yourself up for long-term success.

Building Recovery into Your Routine

1. **Strategic Rest Days**

   - **Planning Rest Days**: Discuss the importance of scheduling rest days in your weekly workout routine. Highlight how strategically placing rest days can prevent burnout and allow muscles to repair and grow.
   - **Active Rest**: Suggest incorporating light activities on rest days, such as walking or yoga, to promote blood flow without straining the body.

2. **Listening to Your Body**

   - **Recognizing Signs of Overtraining**: Detail the common signs of overtraining, such as prolonged fatigue, irritability, decreased performance, and increased susceptibility to injuries. Emphasize the need to listen to these signals and adjust training accordingly.
   - **When to Pull Back**: Provide guidance on how to determine when it's necessary to reduce workout intensity or volume. Encourage readers to take proactive steps to prevent burnout and prioritize long-term health over short-term gains.

3. **Recovery Tools**

   - **Massage Guns**: Explain how massage guns can aid in muscle recovery by increasing blood flow, reducing soreness, and enhancing flexibility. Include tips on effective usage.

- o **Cold Baths**: Discuss the benefits of cold baths or ice baths for reducing inflammation and speeding up recovery post-workout, along with considerations for those with heart conditions.
- o **Foam Rollers and Other Techniques**: Briefly mention foam rolling and other recovery techniques (like stretching and mobility work) that can help alleviate muscle tension and promote recovery.

VII. Conclusion: Recovery as a Non-Negotiable Component

1. Recovery is Non-Negotiable

- o **Essential for Results**: Reinforce that recovery is not just an optional part of fitness; it is a critical component for achieving optimal results. Without proper recovery, the efforts invested in workouts can lead to setbacks, diminished performance, and injuries.
- o **Preventing Burnout and Injury**: Highlight the dangers of neglecting recovery, including burnout, chronic fatigue, and increased risk of injury, which can derail progress and impede reaching fitness goals.

2. Sustainable Progress

- o **Long-Term Success**: Emphasize that making recovery a priority fosters a sustainable approach to fitness. It's not just about immediate gains; it's about establishing a foundation for lasting health, better fat loss, and muscle gain.
- o **A Holistic Approach**: Stress the importance of viewing recovery as an integral part of a comprehensive fitness strategy. This mindset can enhance motivation, adherence, and overall success in achieving personal fitness goals.

3. The Path Ahead

- o **Integrating Recovery**: Encourage readers to evaluate their current routines and consciously incorporate the recovery strategies discussed throughout the chapter. Recognize that even small adjustments can lead to significant improvements in performance and well-being.
- o **Patience is Key**: Conclude by emphasizing that fitness is a journey requiring patience and perseverance. A commitment to recovery not only enhances physical performance but also nurtures a healthier, more balanced lifestyle.

Chapter 5: Keeping It Simple: How to Stay Consistent

I. Introduction to Consistency

The Importance of Consistency

Consistency is the cornerstone of achieving fitness and weight loss goals. It goes beyond merely showing up for workouts; it encompasses maintaining a balanced approach to nutrition and recovery. When we commit to consistent actions, no matter how small, we build momentum over time, allowing us to make significant progress. Each step taken regularly contributes to lasting change, both physically and mentally.

While quick fixes may provide temporary results, true transformation demands a long-term commitment. Understanding the difference between short-term diets and sustainable lifestyle changes is crucial. Consistent effort not only helps us achieve our goals but also aids in maintaining them, creating a healthier relationship with fitness and well-being.

Beyond the physical aspect, consistency has profound psychological benefits. Establishing and adhering to a routine enhances mental resilience. When we see progress from our consistent efforts, it boosts our confidence, reduces anxiety about our journey, and fosters a positive mindset. It reminds us that persistence is key; every small victory counts.

Simplicity in Approach

In the quest for consistency, simplicity emerges as a powerful ally. Overcomplicating our routines or diets can lead to frustration and burnout. When we simplify our habits, we can focus on what truly matters without feeling overwhelmed by the details.

Creating manageable habits is essential. Rather than overhauling our entire lifestyle, starting with small changes can be incredibly effective. For instance, adding more vegetables to meals or committing to a short walk after dinner can lay the foundation for healthier living. These small shifts are not only easier to integrate into daily life but also set the stage for more significant changes over time.

Simplicity also plays a crucial role in reducing decision fatigue, a common barrier to consistency. When our plans are straightforward, we're less likely to hesitate or make unhealthy choices due to indecision. Simple meal plans, easy-to-follow workout routines, and clear habit trackers can make it easier to stay on track without second-guessing ourselves.

Consider the 80/20 principle, which suggests focusing on the 20% of actions that yield 80% of the results. By concentrating on a few key habits—like regular exercise and balanced nutrition —we can achieve most of our desired outcomes without getting bogged down in unnecessary details. This approach allows us to maintain focus and energy for the aspects of our journey that truly matter.

As we move through this chapter, we'll delve deeper into building sustainable habits, overcoming plateaus, and tracking progress in a way that emphasizes simplicity. With a solid understanding of consistency and a simplified approach, you'll be well-equipped to navigate your fitness journey effectively.

Building Sustainable Habits

The Habit Loop

Understanding the components of habit formation is essential for building sustainable habits. The **habit loop** consists of three key elements:

- **Cue:** This is the trigger that initiates your habit. For instance, after a long day at work, you might feel tired and look for a quick source of comfort. Recognizing this cue is the first step in modifying your behavior.

- **Routine:** The routine is the behavior itself—what you do in response to the cue. In my case, hitting the gym has become a non-negotiable part of my daily routine. After finishing work at 4 PM, I head straight to the gym. This decision removes any "ifs" or doubts; it's a commitment I've made to myself. If I miss a session, I don't beat myself up too much, but I definitely feel the urge to get back on track. The satisfaction and energy I gain from working out reinforce this habit.

- **Reward:** Every habit loop ends with a reward, which reinforces the behavior. The endorphins released after a good workout provide a natural high that makes it easier to keep returning to the gym. This reward reinforces the habit and keeps you motivated to continue.

Start Small

When trying to build new habits, starting small is crucial. Gradual changes are more sustainable and less overwhelming. For example, instead of overhauling your entire diet, focus on replacing one unhealthy snack with a healthier option. You don't have to cut everything out immediately. Moderation is key.

Tracking what you eat can be incredibly enlightening. Initially, you might indulge in pizza or other comfort foods but start to notice how they affect your energy levels. By keeping a food diary or using an app, you can visually see patterns in your eating habits. This awareness can motivate you to make better choices without feeling deprived.

Habit Stacking

Habit stacking involves pairing a new habit with an existing one, making it easier to integrate into your daily life. For instance, if you're already going to the gym regularly, you might pair that with meal prepping on Sundays. This way, the workout becomes a cue for you to prepare healthy meals, reinforcing both habits simultaneously.

Consider adding a quick stretching routine after your workouts. This additional habit can improve your flexibility and overall recovery. By stacking habits, you create a synergistic effect, making it easier to adhere to your fitness and nutrition goals.

Environmental Design

Your environment plays a significant role in supporting your habits. **Environmental design** means creating a space that encourages healthy choices. Here are some practical tips:

- **Meal Prep**: Dedicate some time on weekends to prepare meals for the week ahead. This not only saves time but also ensures you have nutritious options readily available, reducing the temptation for takeout.

- **Visibility of Healthy Foods**: Keep healthy snacks like fruits, nuts, or yogurt in plain sight. If they're visible, you're more likely to grab them instead of reaching for junk food hidden away.

- **Workout Gear**: Lay out your gym clothes the night before. When you see them first thing in the morning, it serves as a visual cue to get moving.

- **Motivational Reminders**: Place motivational quotes or images of your fitness goals around your living space. These visual reminders can reinforce your commitment and keep you focused.

Conclusion

Building sustainable habits is a journey that requires patience and dedication. Acknowledge that setbacks are a natural part of the process; they don't mean failure. The key is to stay consistent and committed to your goals. Remember, every small change contributes to lasting transformation. By focusing on creating simple, manageable habits, you'll set yourself up for long-term success in your fitness and nutrition journey.

Avoiding Plateaus

Understanding Plateaus

In fitness and weight loss, a **plateau** refers to a period of little to no progress despite continued effort in training and nutrition. It's a frustrating experience that can happen to anyone, regardless of their experience level. Plateaus are not just common; they are an **inevitable part of the journey**. In fact, it's illogical to expect continuous progress without interruption. Imagine if we were able to continuously put on muscle without any limits; we would end up as mountains! Our bodies need time to adapt, recover, and recalibrate.

Plateaus occur for several reasons, including:

- **Adaptation**: Your body is incredibly efficient and quickly adapts to the stresses you place on it. When you perform the same workouts repeatedly, your muscles become accustomed to the routine, leading to diminished returns in strength and fat loss.

- **Nutritional Factors**: If your caloric intake doesn't align with your goals, you may find that your body is not getting the fuel it needs to continue making progress. Consuming the same macronutrient distribution over time can lead to stagnation.

- **Recovery Issues**: Insufficient recovery can impede progress. If you're not allowing your body adequate time to rest and recover, it may not respond optimally to your training.

Understanding that plateaus are a natural and necessary aspect of fitness can help you maintain perspective and motivate you to make the necessary adjustments. They serve as a reminder that your body is working hard to adapt to the challenges you present it, and they provide an opportunity to reassess and refine your approach. Rather than viewing plateaus as setbacks, consider them as critical moments for growth and reflection on your fitness journey.

Strategies to Break Through Plateaus

Varying Workouts

One of the most effective ways to break through a plateau is by **varying your workouts**. Here are some practical strategies:

- **Change Your Exercises**: Rotate in new exercises that target the same muscle groups. If you usually bench press, try incline or decline presses, or even switch to dumbbells instead of barbells. This change can stimulate muscle growth and strength.

- **Modify Repetition Ranges**: Adjust the number of reps and sets. If you typically perform 3 sets of 10 reps, switch to 4 sets of 6-8 reps or 2 sets of 15-20 reps. Altering these variables can challenge your muscles differently and promote growth.

- **Incorporate Different Training Styles**: Try adding different types of training, such as high-intensity interval training (HIIT), circuit training, or functional movements. These variations can shock your body and push past plateaus.

Varying Workouts: Adjusting your workout plan when it feels like it has maximized its effectiveness can challenge your body and stimulate progress. Personally, if I notice that my nutrition and recovery are on point but I'm still not seeing results, I rotate between different workout plans. For instance, after focusing heavily on strength training, I switch to a program with higher volume and repetitions for hypertrophy. Not only does this keep my training effective, but it also adds an element of fun—sometimes, it's just nice to switch things up because sticking to the same routine can get monotonous!

Adjusting Nutrition

Sometimes, the solution to a plateau lies in your nutrition. Consider these adjustments:

- **Reassess Your Caloric Intake**: If you've been following the same caloric intake for an extended period, your metabolism may have adapted, which can hinder progress. For example, if you started with a 500-calorie deficit and have lost weight, the math changes: your body now requires fewer calories to maintain its new weight. This means that you are no longer in a deficit of 500 calories. To continue losing weight, you may need to decrease your caloric intake further. Regularly reassessing your caloric needs is essential to ensure you stay on track and create an effective plan for ongoing weight loss.

- **Modify Macronutrient Ratios**: Consider adjusting the ratio of proteins, fats, and carbohydrates. Increasing protein intake can be particularly beneficial when in a caloric deficit, as it helps preserve lean muscle mass and aids recovery. Alternatively, lowering carbohydrate intake for a period can prompt your body to utilize fat as a fuel source.

- **Track and Reflect**: Use a food diary or app to track your nutrition. Reflecting on your eating habits can highlight areas for improvement or change, such as portion sizes or hidden calories.

Periodization

Periodization is a systematic approach to training that involves cycling through different training phases to prevent stagnation. It can be broken down into three main phases:

- **Macrocycle**: This is the overall training plan that spans several months to a year, focusing on long-term goals.

- **Mesocycle**: Each macrocycle consists of several mesocycles, typically lasting a few weeks to a few months. Each mesocycle can focus on specific goals, such as strength building, hypertrophy, or endurance.

- **Microcycle**: This is the smallest training cycle, often lasting a week. Within each microcycle, you can vary intensity, volume, and exercises to keep your body challenged.

By strategically planning your workouts with periodization, you allow your body to adapt to new stresses and reduce the risk of plateaus. This structured approach promotes continuous progress, making it easier to maintain motivation and achieve your goals.

Conclusion

Plateaus are a natural part of the fitness journey, but they don't have to be permanent. By understanding what causes plateaus and implementing strategies to overcome them—such as varying workouts, adjusting nutrition, and utilizing periodization—you can keep your progress on track. Remember, persistence is key, and with the right mindset and strategies, you can continue to make strides toward your fitness and weight loss goals. While all these strategies may initially seem overwhelming, it's essential to remember that with time and practice, they will start to fall into place. Consistency is key, and as you integrate these habits into your daily routine, they will become second nature. Trust the process, and allow yourself the patience to adapt and grow.

Tracking Progress Effectively

Different Metrics for Tracking:

- **Beyond the Scale:**
  Relying solely on the scale can be misleading and disheartening, especially as body composition changes. Consider alternative measures of progress, such as:
    - **Body Measurements:** Regularly measure key areas like waist, hips, chest, arms, and legs. Changes in these measurements can provide a clearer picture of your progress, even when the scale doesn't budge.
    - **How Clothes Fit:** Notice how your clothes feel and fit over time. This can be a more relatable indicator of progress, as clothes becoming looser often reflects fat loss and muscle gain.
    - **Performance Metrics:** Track improvements in your workouts, such as lifting heavier weights, completing more reps, or increasing endurance in cardio activities. These gains signify strength and fitness improvements, regardless of what the scale says.
    - **The Mirror:** Using the mirror as a tracking tool can be a powerful way to assess your physical progress. Often, changes in muscle definition, body composition, and overall appearance may not immediately show on the scale. By regularly checking your reflection, you can visually appreciate the improvements in your physique, such as increased muscle tone or a slimmer waistline. This can boost your motivation and help you recognize that progress comes in many forms, beyond just the numbers.

Use of Journals or Apps:

- **Recommended Tools:**
  Keeping track of your progress is vital for accountability and motivation. Consider the following tools:
    - **Workout Journals:** A simple notebook or a digital app can help log your workouts, sets, reps, and weights. This tracking helps you see your improvements over time and adjust your routine as needed.
    - **Nutrition Tracking Apps:** Apps like MyFitnessPal, Cronometer or Lifesum can help monitor your food intake, ensuring you meet your nutritional goals while being mindful of calories and macronutrients.
    - **Mood and Energy Tracking:** Documenting your feelings and energy levels can provide insight into how your workouts and nutrition impact your overall well-being.

Setting Realistic Goals:

- **The SMART Approach:**
  Setting realistic and achievable goals is crucial for long-term success. Consider the SMART framework:
    - **Specific:** Clearly define what you want to achieve. Instead of saying "I want to lose weight," specify "I want to lose 10 pounds in the next three months."
    - **Measurable:** Ensure that your goals can be tracked. For instance, measure your body weight, body fat percentage, or the number of workouts completed.
    - **Achievable:** Set goals that are challenging yet attainable. Consider your current lifestyle, commitments, and physical condition to create realistic expectations.
    - **Relevant:** Your goals should align with your overall objectives and values. Ensure they are meaningful to you and will motivate you to stay consistent.
    - **Time-bound:** Establish a deadline for your goals. Setting a timeframe creates urgency and encourages you to stay focused and accountable.

Progress You Can See and Feel

Tracking progress might seem detailed, but it's essential for staying motivated and recognizing how far you've come. While the scale can be one measure, looking at other markers—like your strength, energy levels, and the changes you see in the mirror—gives a more complete view of your progress. Using apps, journals, or simply taking note of how your clothes fit helps keep you on track without obsessing over one metric. As you set **SMART goals** and follow your journey, you'll start seeing how each small step and adjustment contributes to your bigger vision, making the process rewarding and sustainable.

The Role of Mindset in Consistency

Growth vs. Fixed Mindset

Your mindset can determine how you experience challenges, setbacks, and progress in any fitness journey. A growth mindset helps you view each setback or plateau as a stepping stone rather than a roadblock. People with a growth mindset tend to embrace learning and see skills as something to be developed, whereas those with a fixed mindset might see setbacks as proof of their limitations. Think about your fitness routine: there will be times when results come slower than you'd like or when a new exercise feels impossible. Instead of thinking, "I can't do this," try shifting to "I can't do this yet." This approach makes you more adaptable and encourages you to push through rough patches rather than giving up.

Examples of Growth Mindset in Action

- **Learning from Plateaus**: If you hit a plateau, a growth mindset prompts you to try new strategies—adjusting nutrition, modifying workouts, or adding rest days—instead of giving up or sticking to what no longer works.
- **Skill Development**: Even with exercises that seem challenging (like deadlifts or pull-ups), a growth mindset helps you focus on gradual improvement. Rather than expecting instant mastery, each small gain—like adding an extra rep or improving form—is a success that motivates you to keep going.
- **Mindset in Recovery**: Recovery is just as essential as the work itself. Shifting your view of recovery days from "time wasted" to "growth time" strengthens your overall approach, keeping you focused on the long term.

Dealing with Setbacks

Setbacks are inevitable, but it's how you handle them that makes the difference. These moments often reveal weaknesses, either in approach or mindset, and highlight what needs improvement. If a stressful week at work keeps you from the gym, for example, a fixed mindset might lead you to feel like a failure. Instead, take this moment to reflect on what went wrong and why. Use this reflection to make small adjustments—maybe a shorter workout or quick home routine—that help you bounce back rather than derail entirely.

Practical Tips for Handling Setbacks

- **Find the Lesson**: Each setback can be a learning experience. If you miss a workout, ask yourself what got in the way and whether there's something you can change. Did you over-schedule, or do you need a backup plan for busy days?
- **Stay Accountable**: Checking in with yourself regularly can help. This could mean using a journal or an app where you track your workouts and note how you feel. Seeing your progress—even if it's not linear—reminds you that every step counts.
- **Celebrate Small Wins**: Setbacks are easier to manage if you recognize the small wins along the way. Didn't make it to the gym? Consider that you still stuck to healthy nutrition or managed to get more steps in. Acknowledging small victories helps you feel accomplished and keeps you moving forward.

Staying Consistent During Challenges

When challenges arise, remind yourself why you started. Think back to the motivation that led you to pursue fitness or weight loss and the goals you're working toward. Developing strategies to stay engaged—whether it's planning workouts with friends, adjusting your routine, or setting small weekly targets—gives you renewed energy and keeps things interesting.

Making Consistency Enjoyable

Finding Enjoyment in the Process

The key to long-term success is making the journey enjoyable, so it feels less like a chore and more like a fulfilling part of life. Choosing workouts and foods that you actually look forward to can transform how you feel about consistency. If you're someone who dreads the gym, try experimenting with different forms of movement until you find one that clicks—anything from hiking, swimming, or dance classes to boxing or functional training can make working out feel like play rather than work. The goal is to find activities you love that also contribute to your fitness.

Similarly, focusing on foods that nourish you *and* that you enjoy makes sticking to your nutrition plan easier. Instead of forcing yourself to eat "diet" foods you don't like, try experimenting with spices, flavors, and ingredients that you're drawn to. Making enjoyable choices increases the likelihood that you'll stay consistent without feeling deprived, which ultimately makes the journey a positive experience.

Quick Tips for Enjoying the Process

- **Celebrate Small Milestones**: Setting mini-goals—like mastering a new exercise, achieving performance milestones, or noticing small changes in your physique—gives you steady, achievable targets to celebrate along the way. These mini-goals keep things exciting and reinforce the larger journey. For example, setting a goal like "I want to bench 200 pounds in 1-2 years" can keep you motivated with your eyes on the prize. This approach lets you break down big goals into manageable steps, helping you stay committed while seeing measurable progress, one milestone at a time.
- **Switch Things Up**: Adding variety to your routine can prevent boredom. Rotate through different workout styles, or introduce new recipes or cuisines. Small changes keep things fresh and challenging.
- **Make Time for Rewards**: Don't underestimate the power of a good post-workout ritual—whether it's treating yourself to a favorite smoothie, a relaxing stretch session, or simply taking a moment to reflect on your progress. Building a reward system reinforces the habit and makes the entire process more enjoyable. And hey, if you've really earned it and stayed consistent, go ahead and indulge a bit! Get a pizza, grab a beer or two, and savor the balance. Just remember that consistency, paired with the occasional reward, keeps the journey sustainable and rewarding in the long run.

Social Support

Finding a support system or community can make a world of difference, both for accountability and for enjoyment. Having people around who understand and support your goals gives you a source of encouragement on tough days and a group to celebrate with on good ones. Joining a fitness class, teaming up with a gym buddy, or even participating in an online fitness group can help build a sense of connection and motivation. People who share similar goals will understand your challenges and wins, and they can offer insights that help you along the way.

Ideas for Building a Support System

- **Workout Partners**: Find someone with similar fitness goals to join you in workouts. Having a workout partner not only makes exercise more enjoyable but also adds a level of accountability—knowing someone else is counting on you makes it harder to skip workouts. And if getting a friend to join you seems challenging, don't worry. Personally, I've trained with friends only once or twice. My best motivation came from people I met in the gym itself—those who naturally became workout partners over time, sharing the same dedication. Real workout partners are often those who push you by simply being there and sharing the same commitment, turning the gym into a space where motivation thrives.
- **Community Classes**: Participating in group fitness sessions can foster camaraderie and add a layer of friendly competition, often helping you push harder than you might on your own. These classes bring something extra to the experience—you'll meet people who have been attending for years, and others who, like you, are just starting out. There are always new faces and someone sharing the same goals as you. Group sessions create a motivating atmosphere where each person's energy lifts the others, turning fitness into a shared journey rather than a solo pursuit.
- **Online Groups and Challenges**: Many online communities provide motivation through shared progress, recipes, fitness tips, and daily encouragement. Being part of a virtual community can be just as supportive as having people around in real life. There's a huge variety of forums and groups out there, filled with people on similar fitness journeys, sharing everything from personal milestones to fun, relatable stories. Jumping into one of these communities can add a great sense of camaraderie and a boost of inspiration whenever you need it—plus, it's a fun way to stay connected and motivated.

VII. Conclusion: Simplifying Your Journey

Embracing Simplicity as a Path to Success

Throughout this book, you've seen how critical consistency and simplicity are to reaching your fitness goals. It might feel overwhelming at first—tracking habits, adjusting routines, staying mindful of nutrition. But just like learning to drive a stick shift, where throttle, clutch, and gear shifting all seem chaotic in the beginning, the steps in this journey will become second nature with time. Each small action will start to flow naturally into the next until they're just part of your routine.

Commitment to the Process

Staying committed is key. Every small step counts, and even when it feels complicated, remember that mastery comes with time and patience. Don't overthink or overcomplicate things—take it day by day. Progress will come naturally as each habit falls into place, supporting you on a path that's sustainable and rewarding. You're building something lasting here, one small step at a time.

Chapter 6: Truth in Action: Real Results Without the Lies

I. Introduction

In the world of fitness, where information is abundant and often conflicting, authenticity stands as a beacon for anyone embarking on their health journey. The path to achieving fitness goals is rarely linear; it is filled with ups and downs, successes and setbacks. Yet, it's these genuine experiences that resonate most deeply, showcasing the real struggles and triumphs that many face.

This chapter is dedicated to celebrating the power of authenticity in fitness journeys. By sharing compelling case studies and personal stories, we aim to inspire and motivate you. These narratives not only highlight the diverse paths individuals have taken but also underscore the common threads of resilience, determination, and perseverance.

In a society often inundated with unrealistic portrayals of health and fitness, it's crucial to remind ourselves that real progress comes from honest efforts. Whether you're just starting or are well on your way, the stories shared in this chapter will provide you with relatable examples of what it means to chase your goals genuinely.

Let's dive into these journeys, learn from them, and find inspiration in the truth of real results —because the only lies we should leave behind are those that tell us success comes without hard work, commitment, and authenticity.

Case Studies

Note on Case Studies

In the following case studies, the names and identifying details of individuals have been changed to protect their privacy. While the stories shared are based on real experiences, the focus is on their journeys and the strategies they employed to achieve their fitness goals. These narratives aim to inspire and motivate readers by illustrating the power of authenticity in the pursuit of health and wellness.

Case Study 1: John's Transformation

Profile

- **Name**: John
- **Age**: 33
- **Starting Weight**: 220 lbs
- **End Weight:** 145 lbs (approximately 66 kg)
- **Fitness Level**: Regular gym-goer but lacked intensity and focus

Challenges Faced

John faced several challenges throughout his journey. Known as a "party freak," he often overindulged in alcohol and made extremely poor food choices. Although he was a regular gym-goer, his lack of intensity and focus resulted in stagnation while others around him thrived. It was frustrating to see his lack of progress, which felt obvious to me, but remained a mystery to him.

Strategies Used

To combat his challenges, John implemented several key strategies:

- **Nutrition**: I recommended that he start tracking everything he drank and ate. The results were eye-opening; some days he consumed over 5,000 kcal, while on others, he barely hit 1,000 kcal. This awareness helped him realize the extent of his eating habits. Instead of drastic dieting, he focused on portion control and started incorporating more whole foods like fruits, vegetables, and lean proteins. He also replaced regular burgers and pizza with healthier options.

- **Workouts**: Initially, his workouts were lackluster—without challenging lifts or ambition, it was just a place he visited for 45 minutes before leaving. With the tools I provided, I encouraged him to be more intentional with his training. He began to embrace low-impact cardio like walking and cycling, gradually increasing the intensity, and eventually incorporated strength training into his routine three times a week.

- **Mindset Shifts**: John worked on changing his mindset by setting realistic, short-term goals. Instead of fixating solely on weight loss, he celebrated non-scale victories such as improved endurance and increased energy levels. Although he couldn't give up drinking entirely, he learned to moderate his intake and make better choices.

Results

Over 12 months, John lost a total of 75 lbs. The transformation was remarkable—he was no longer the same person I had known for years. He reported increased energy, improved self-esteem, and a newfound passion for exercise. Now, he regularly participates in community fitness events and has built lasting friendships in the gym.

Case Study 2: Tim's Journey to Health

Profile

- **Age:** 45
- **Starting Weight:** 300 lbs (approximately 136 kg)
- **End Weight:** 212 lbs (approximately 96 kg)
- **Fitness Level:** Inactive, with a history of high blood pressure and joint pain

Challenges Faced

Tim's journey was marked by significant health concerns, including high blood pressure and joint pain, which made physical activity particularly challenging. He struggled with motivation, feeling discouraged by previous failed attempts at weight loss. Additionally, he fell victim to expensive fad trends that promised quick results but left him feeling frustrated and disillusioned. This went on for years! Tim regularly complained that nothing seemed to work for losing weight, and the situation escalated to a heart attack and episodes of shortness of breath.

Strategies Used

To finally turn his life around, Tim adopted a comprehensive approach:

- **Nutrition:** He took charge of his own nutrition, developing a balanced meal plan focused on heart-healthy foods. Tim significantly reduced his sodium intake and increased his consumption of whole grains, fruits, and vegetables, moving away from the costly fad diets that had previously let him down.

- **Workouts:** Tim preferred walking and jogging in the forest, as he didn't enjoy the gym environment. He started with gentle walks and gradually increased his pace, incorporating jogging into his routine as he became more comfortable.

- **Mindset Shifts:** After suffering a heart attack, Tim finally faced the harsh reality of his situation. Is that what it takes for people to stop lying to themselves? The wake-up call pushed him to reassess his habits and choices. He began to keep a journal to track his progress and reflect on his feelings, helping him maintain motivation through challenging days. Although he had previously insisted he wasn't eating a lot, the truth became undeniable once he started tracking his intake. The verdict? Not good.

Results

After one year, Tim achieved an impressive weight loss of **88 lbs (approximately 40 kg)**! His blood pressure stabilized, and he reported feeling more energetic and engaged in life. The heart attack served as a crucial turning point, leading him to embrace a healthier lifestyle that he had long resisted. Tim's newfound enthusiasm for walking and jogging allowed him to enjoy the outdoors while improving his overall health and well-being.

Tim is a great dude! An awesome dude! But do not be like Tim! Don't wait for something life-threatening to make the necessary choices. Take action now to prioritize your health and well-being.

Case Study 3: Emilio's Fitness Evolution
Profile

- **Age:** 23
- **Starting Weight:** 150 lbs
- **End Weight:** 167 lbs
- **Fitness Level:** Regular exerciser but with no definable muscle mass; described as "skinny fat."

Challenges Faced

Emilio struggled with a lack of muscle definition and often found himself in a "yo-yo" dieting cycle. He tried various trends but lacked a clear strategy for building muscle, which left him frustrated with his body composition. Additionally, he often underestimated his caloric needs, believing he was consuming enough to support muscle growth while actually maintaining a deficit.

His focus on aesthetics sometimes overshadowed the importance of a comprehensive fitness approach, leading him to prioritize quick fixes over sustainable methods. He frequently rationalized setbacks, convincing himself that he was doing better than he actually was, and avoided tracking his intake and workouts, which prevented him from holding himself accountable. This cycle of self-deception hindered his progress and kept him from recognizing the effort required for meaningful change.

Strategies Used

To create a sustainable fitness journey, Emilio made several significant adjustments:

- **Nutrition:** He focused on increasing his protein intake, adjusting his nutrition to ensure he was fueling his body appropriately for muscle growth. Emilio adopted a flexible eating approach, maintaining a smaller calorie deficit of around 200 calories, allowing him to still enjoy food while making progress.
- **Workouts:** Emilio transitioned from casual exercise to a structured strength training program designed to build muscle mass. He worked with a trainer to learn proper techniques and progressively increase the intensity of his workouts.
- **Mindset Shifts:** He shifted his perspective from solely focusing on aesthetics to prioritizing overall health and muscle development. Emilio learned to embrace the process, understanding that building muscle takes time and consistency.

Results

Over the course of **7-8 months**, Emilio achieved a remarkable transformation, ending at **167 lbs** with a defined physique and visible abs. His body composition improved significantly as he shed the fat that contributed to his "skinny fat" classification, allowing the muscle he built to become more prominent. Emilio now enjoys strength training and is committed to maintaining a balanced and nutritious lifestyle.

overall well-being. Each individual's story reinforces the message that with dedication, authentic strategies, and the right mindset, anyone can achieve their fitness goals.

Collective Insights and Practical Lessons

Each journey in this chapter sheds light on the realities of achieving lasting fitness results, emphasizing that it's never about gimmicks or shortcuts but a commitment to sustainable practices. Here are some universal lessons drawn from John, Tim, and Emilio's experiences that highlight both the challenges and practical strategies anyone can use.

Lessons from the Journey

- **Consistency Over Perfection**
  John, Tim, and Emilio all faced obstacles, from unhealthy habits to physical limitations and lack of muscle definition. Each of their paths required a steady approach that prioritized consistency over drastic measures. For John, tracking his food intake daily

made him aware of his choices without requiring extreme dieting. Tim's commitment to gentle but regular physical activity like walking in the forest kept him consistent even though he had tried many failed approaches before. Emilio's journey highlighted how small, progressive adjustments to his workouts and nutrition helped him move away from restrictive diets and yo-yo cycles.

- **Building Self-Awareness**
  All three individuals struggled initially with seeing the reality of their situation. Whether it was John's high-calorie weekends, Tim's denial of his actual eating habits, or Emilio's focus on ineffective workout routines, self-awareness was a major turning point. The realization of how their daily habits affected their fitness results encouraged them to take ownership of their journey and make mindful decisions.

Breakthrough Moments

- **Embracing Sustainable Changes**
  Each case demonstrates how real change comes from adopting sustainable, not extreme, strategies. John started by moderating his calorie intake rather than cutting it drastically, leading to a 75-pound weight loss over a year. Tim's heart attack served as a wake-up call that motivated him to focus on heart-healthy foods, emphasizing that shortcuts or "fast fixes" can't replace the basics of good nutrition. Emilio's gradual shift to strength training and learning proper techniques allowed him to build the physique he wanted without losing muscle definition to fad dieting.

- **Redefining Goals**
  Transforming goals from simply "losing weight" or "getting ripped" to more meaningful and specific outcomes made the difference in their mindset. For example, instead of just aiming to shed pounds, John celebrated increased energy and endurance as wins. Emilio's focus evolved from superficial aesthetics to overall health and muscle development, a mindset that made his progress more fulfilling and sustainable.

Overcoming Setbacks Together

- **Resilience Strategies**
  Setbacks are part of every fitness journey, and learning to navigate them is essential. John faced the difficulty of balancing social outings and overindulgent habits but found that being mindful and moderating these behaviors was far more realistic than attempting total restriction. Tim learned the hard way that health cannot be taken for

granted, and after his heart attack, he finally committed to maintaining healthier habits. Emilio found it challenging to gain muscle as a "skinny fat" individual, but by sticking to structured training and a slight calorie deficit, he was able to see the progress he had long been chasing.

- **Accountability Tools**
  Each case study emphasized the power of tracking and accountability. Tim found clarity in documenting his daily intake, while Emilio's structured workout plan helped him stay on track and motivated. For John, tracking calories revealed patterns that he was previously blind to, providing the feedback necessary to change course.

Mindset and Consistency

- **Growth Mindset in Fitness**
  The ability to view setbacks as temporary and learn from them was essential for each of these individuals. They each shifted from focusing on quick results to adopting a mindset of long-term improvement. John's emphasis on non-scale victories allowed him to enjoy the journey without getting bogged down by the numbers. Tim's journal became a tool for self-reflection and motivation, helping him stay consistent on tough days. Emilio's mindset evolved as he began to value strength and muscle over scale weight, enabling him to make gains that dieting alone hadn't achieved.

- **Progress, Not Perfection**
  Success doesn't require perfection. Small steps, like John's moderation of alcohol or Tim's switch from fad diets to simple, heart-friendly foods, enabled them to build and maintain healthier habits. Emilio's switch to structured strength training reminded him that visible progress requires time and patience, a reality that often goes unmentioned in the fitness industry.

Final Takeaway: Practical Tips for Your Own Journey

These stories prove that real, sustainable fitness results are accessible to anyone who commits to realistic changes. Just as John, Tim, and Emilio each found their own paths, readers are encouraged to:

1. **Set Realistic Goals**: Start small, focusing on manageable changes that fit your lifestyle.
2. **Embrace Tracking Tools**: Use tools like food journals, workout plans, or a simple notepad to track habits, progress, and setbacks.
3. **Celebrate Non-Scale Victories**: Remember that progress isn't only about weight loss or muscle gains; it's about feeling more energized, healthier, and resilient.

4. **Commit to Consistency**: Change happens with steady effort. Commit to staying consistent, even on days when motivation feels low.

Part IV: Motivational Insights: Real Words from Real Journeys

Rather than just listing mantras, let's focus on a few unfiltered truths and key moments that these individuals faced, leaving readers with real-life takeaways they can hold onto.

Hard Lessons and Realizations

From John:

"I was tired of doing the same thing in the gym and expecting results. It wasn't about a lack of time or energy; I just didn't want it enough to push myself. Once I realized that, everything changed."

John's turning point was recognizing his own lack of commitment. He knew that if he kept going through the motions, he'd never get anywhere. His lesson? Be honest with yourself, stop blaming the program, and start bringing intensity.

From Tim:

"I used to think I wasn't eating that much—until I started tracking. It was like finally seeing the truth after years of denial."

Tim's wake-up call didn't come from any coach or trend but from taking a hard look at his habits. The heart attack may have been a turning point, but the real shift came when he accepted the facts he'd been ignoring. For anyone out there: don't wait for a health scare. Start today by being brutally honest about what's holding you back.

From Emilio:

"I was frustrated that I wasn't getting any bigger, just 'skinnier.' My workouts felt like they weren't paying off. But then I committed to a solid plan, and things slowly—but surely—shifted."

Emilio's journey wasn't a 90-day miracle transformation. He kept pushing even when his progress felt invisible, and eventually, he broke out of the "skinny-fat" cycle. His insight? Stick to the plan long enough to see it work.

Mindset Shifts They Embraced

The one thing each of these people shared was a shift in how they saw the journey itself.

- **Honesty is the Foundation:** John faced the fact that he wasn't bringing his all to his workouts. Tim finally admitted that his eating was out of control. Emilio recognized that he couldn't keep chasing quick fixes. They each embraced the power of honesty and realized it was their path forward.

- **Focus on Showing Up, Not Just the Scale:** Progress isn't always about what the scale says. For each of them, moments of self-respect and accountability meant more than any number. Readers should look at their own goals beyond pounds lost or inches cut and measure success by how often they show up and put in the work.

- **Stop Expecting Perfect Conditions:** There will never be a perfect moment to start or an easy stretch where results happen fast. If you're waiting for that, you're waiting forever. Start where you are, with what you have, and do the best you can. That's what these guys did, and it's what worked.

Encouragement for Readers: A Challenge, Not a Pep Talk

What do all of these cases have in common? **They constantly deceived themselves.** Each of these individuals had moments of denial—whether it was John not acknowledging his lack of intensity in the gym, Tim refusing to admit he was eating more than he thought, or Emilio jumping from one quick fix to another hoping for easy results. The truth is, these deceptions held them back for years.

So here's the challenge: if you're serious about this, stop lying to yourself.

- **Face Your Habits Head-On:** Each of these transformations began when they confronted their habits honestly. If you think you're giving it your all, take a second look. Are you tracking everything? Are you skipping workouts? Self-deception is the fastest way to go nowhere.

- **Patience is Part of the Process:** They all wanted results, and they wanted them fast. But change doesn't happen overnight, and none of them saw drastic progress until they accepted the slow grind and stuck with it. Patience isn't optional—it's mandatory. Real results take time, so focus on consistency, not speed.

- **Consistency Over Perfection:** Each one of them had setbacks, made mistakes, and had off days. But what separated their success from their past failures was consistency. If you can keep showing up, even imperfectly, you're on the right track.

- **Shift Your Mindset from Quick Fixes to Long-Term Habits:** None of them got where they are by following gimmicks or fads. They broke free from that mindset and focused on sustainable habits that could carry them forward. Building real habits may not be flashy, but it's the only way to see lasting results.

Real change takes work, persistence, and honesty. If you can face the truth about your habits and put in the consistent effort, you'll be further along than 90% of people who quit too soon. Stop lying to yourself—just like John, Tim, and Emilio did—and you'll finally be on the path to real progress.

Part V: Conclusion

The case studies of John, Tim, and Emilio illustrate the diverse journeys individuals can take toward achieving their fitness goals. Despite their unique backgrounds and challenges, several key takeaways emerge that are vital for anyone on a similar path:

1. **Self-Awareness is Crucial:** All three individuals had to confront their own habits and recognize the truths they had been avoiding. Whether it was John's overindulgence, Tim's denial of the severity of his health issues, or Emilio's struggle with muscle definition, honesty about their behaviors was the first step toward change.

2. **Consistency and Patience:** Transformation doesn't happen overnight. Each case reflects the importance of being consistent and patient. Real progress often feels slow, but those who endure and stick to their plans see results.

3. **Personal Accountability:** They all took charge of their own journeys. By tracking their nutrition, adjusting their workout routines, and shifting their mindsets, they became proactive in their approaches. This accountability played a significant role in their success.

4. **Embracing the Process**: The stories highlight the importance of enjoying the journey, not just focusing on the destination. Each individual found value in small victories, celebrating non-scale wins like increased energy and endurance.

5. **Rejecting Industry Myths**: All three transformations remind us that quick fixes and fad diets are often misleading. Authentic change comes from understanding what works for your body and lifestyle, not from following trends that promise immediate results.

In conclusion, real success in fitness comes from a steadfast commitment to one's goals. Your journey may look different from others, and that's okay. Remember that the path to genuine transformation is built on honesty, hard work, and a willingness to adapt. By focusing on these principles, you can carve your own path to success without falling victim to the myths that often permeate the fitness industry. Embrace your journey, stay dedicated, and you'll find that real results are within reach.

Chapter 7: The No BS Conclusion

1. Introduction to the Conclusion

I know some of you might have flipped through certain parts of this book, scanning for what felt like the "big pages" and diving right into sections that seemed to promise quick answers. I understand—sometimes we all look for shortcuts. But here's the truth: *The No BS Way* wasn't written for shortcuts. It's about giving you the real, grounded approach to weight loss and fitness that doesn't rely on hype or industry myths. This isn't a place for gimmicks; it's about giving you the tools to make actual, lasting changes.

So, while I strongly recommend taking the time to read through the whole book, following each chapter in sequence to grasp the full strategy, I also respect your time. And because I want you to walk away with practical steps you can use right now, this conclusion chapter will serve as your "TL;DR." Think of it as a no-nonsense summary, the essential principles without the fluff, focused on what really matters.

Here, we'll review the foundational ideas you need to succeed, the main strategies you can implement starting today, and the hard truths about consistency, accountability, and discipline. This isn't just a recap; it's a reminder of what it takes to turn ambition into action and goals into achievements.

So let's break it down. This is your No BS guide to weight loss, wrapped up in one chapter. Every step in this book has been about putting you in control—no more guessing, no more frustration, just clarity on what really works. Here's what you need to take away from this journey.

Key Takeaways

Core Principles: The Foundations of Real Weight Loss

Throughout this book, we've broken down weight loss into simple, actionable steps. There's no magic formula here—just solid, time-tested principles that get results. Here are the core pillars:

Calorie Tracking: Your Baseline to Control and Awareness

Tracking your calories is more than just logging numbers; it's the foundation of taking control over what you put into your body. By tracking your intake, you're making sure you're in the driver's seat rather than letting random eating patterns control your results. Here's a practical breakdown on how to start tracking calories and turn it into an essential part of your routine:

1. **Choose Your Tools**: Begin by picking a calorie-tracking app that makes the process easy and accurate. Some popular, user-friendly options include:

   - **MyFitnessPal**: One of the most widely used apps for calorie counting, MyFitnessPal has a massive food database and offers easy barcode scanning for packaged foods.
   - **Lose It!**: Known for its intuitive interface, Lose It! is great for beginners and helps you set personal goals.
   - **Cronometer**: If you're after precision, Cronometer is excellent as it tracks micronutrients (vitamins and minerals) alongside calories.
   - **Yazio**: This app combines tracking with meal planning, providing recipe ideas to help you stay within your target calories.
   - **Apple Health & Samsung Health**: Both of these come pre-installed on iPhones and Samsung devices and allow for integration with various food-logging apps.

2. **Set a Target**: Before logging anything, you'll want a daily calorie target. Many tracking apps have built-in calculators based on your age, weight, gender, activity level, and goals (weight loss, maintenance, or muscle gain). These calculators provide a baseline number, but be prepared to adjust based on your weekly progress.

3. **Log Consistently**: Make tracking a habit by logging every meal, snack, and even drinks with calories. The more consistent you are, the more reliable the insights:

   - **Scan Barcodes**: When eating packaged foods, use your app's barcode scanner to instantly input calories and other nutritional info.
   - **Estimate Portions**: For home-cooked meals, weigh your portions or use visual estimations (e.g., a palm-sized portion for protein, a fist-sized portion for carbs).
   - **Track Dining Out**: When eating out, look up similar dishes in your app's database to get an approximate calorie count. Some chain restaurants also have calorie information on their websites or menus.

4. **Understand Macronutrient Balance**: Beyond calorie counting, tracking macronutrients (proteins, carbs, and fats) helps you see if you're meeting the right

balance for your body composition goals. Most apps will automatically break down your macronutrient intake:

- o **For Weight Loss**: Aim for a higher protein intake to preserve muscle while in a calorie deficit.
- o **For Muscle Gain**: Increase protein, along with carbohydrates, to fuel workouts and promote growth.
- o **For Maintenance**: Keep a balance that matches your activity levels, focusing on nutrient-dense foods.

5. **Review and Adjust**: Weekly reviews allow you to gauge your progress and make adjustments. If your weight or measurements aren't moving in the right direction, consider recalibrating your calorie intake by 5-10%:

- o **Plateau?**: If you're not seeing any change after a few weeks, slightly reduce or increase your intake based on your goals.
- o **Overcoming Cravings**: Tracking lets you identify high-calorie foods that might be causing spikes, helping you swap them out for filling, nutrient-dense alternatives.

6. **Leverage Insights to Improve**: After a few weeks, look back at your entries. Notice any patterns? Maybe certain days you tend to overeat, or you're not getting enough protein. Use these insights to tweak your diet and build a sustainable eating pattern:

- o **Energy Dips**: If you find yourself low on energy at certain times, check if you're under-consuming carbs or skipping meals.
- o **Stress Eating**: Identify days or situations that lead to overeating and plan alternative strategies for coping with stress.

7. **Hold Yourself Accountable**: Calorie tracking is not just about food—it's about building self-awareness and accountability. Think of each entry as a commitment to your goals. Over time, this practice becomes second nature and helps you make better food choices automatically.

Physical Activity: A Key Component of Weight Loss and Wellness

Incorporating regular physical activity into your routine is essential for achieving weight loss and maintaining overall health. Here are some important points to consider:

1. **Strength Training:** Aim to include strength training exercises at least 2-3 times a week. This helps build muscle, which boosts your metabolism and supports fat loss.

2. **Cardiovascular Exercise:** Engage in cardiovascular activities like running, cycling, or swimming for at least 150 minutes per week. This enhances heart health, burns calories, and improves endurance.

3. **Flexibility and Mobility:** Don't forget to incorporate flexibility and mobility exercises, such as stretching or yoga. These improve range of motion, reduce injury risk, and aid recovery.

4. **Alternative Activities:** If the gym isn't your scene, don't worry! Consider walking, jogging, dancing, or participating in group sports. The key is to find activities that you enjoy, making it easier to stay consistent.

5. **Stay Active Daily:** Look for opportunities to be active throughout your day. Simple changes like taking the stairs, walking instead of driving short distances, or doing household chores can significantly increase your overall activity level.

Remember, the goal is to create a sustainable routine that keeps you moving and engaged. Whether it's through structured workout plans in this book or enjoyable physical activities outside the gym, find what works for you and stick with it for lasting results.

Mastering Portion Control

For those of you who find calorie tracking tedious, portion control is the practical, "on-the-go" alternative. It's about tuning into your body's signals and respecting its limits. By adopting portion control, you can make a significant impact on your health and weight management without the need for constant calorie counting. Here's how to implement it effectively:

1. **Listen to Your Body**: Become attuned to your hunger and fullness cues. Start by asking yourself if you're truly hungry before reaching for a snack or meal. Pay attention to how your body feels throughout your meal—stop eating when you feel comfortably satisfied, not stuffed.

2. **Balance Your Plate**: Aim for a balanced plate that consists of:

    o **Half Vegetables**: Fill half your plate with a variety of colorful vegetables. They are low in calories and high in nutrients, helping you feel full.
    o **One Quarter Protein**: Choose lean proteins like chicken, fish, beans, or tofu to support muscle repair and overall health.
    o **One Quarter Carbohydrates**: Include whole grains or starchy vegetables in moderation. This provides energy without overloading on calories.

3. **Use Visual Cues**: Familiarize yourself with standard serving sizes using your hands as a guide. For example:

    o A serving of meat is about the size of your palm.
    o A serving of grains is roughly the size of a cupped hand.
    o Fruits and starchy vegetables should fit within a fist.

4. **Mindful Eating Practices**: Take time to enjoy your food. Chew slowly, savor the flavors, and minimize distractions like screens. This practice helps you appreciate your meals and recognize when you've had enough.

5. **Plan and Prep**: Consider meal prepping to control portions better. When you prepare your meals in advance, you can portion out servings, making it easier to stick to appropriate amounts.

6. **Stay Flexible**: Life can be unpredictable, and some days you may need larger or smaller portions based on your activity level. Don't stress about being perfect; listen to your body and adjust accordingly.

7. **Practice Regularly**: Like any skill, mastering portion control takes practice. Keep refining your approach until it feels natural.

By integrating portion control into your daily routine, you can enjoy a variety of foods, satisfy your cravings, and maintain a healthy lifestyle without the constraints of strict calorie tracking. Embrace this simple yet powerful method to help you achieve your weight loss goals and foster a positive relationship with food. Remember, it's about progress, not perfection.

Mindset Shifts: Building the Mental Strength for Real Results

This title emphasizes the foundational role mindset plays in transforming your body and reaching your fitness goals by highlighting that mental resilience and focus are crucial for real, sustainable change. It sets the stage for discussing how lasting success is built on consistency, honesty, and discipline.

- **Accountability**: One of the biggest stumbling blocks is a failure to stay accountable. Skipping the gym, "forgetting" to track calories, or making excuses to eat poorly are common habits that sabotage progress. Being accountable means not letting yourself off the hook or downplaying poor choices. It's about owning up to mistakes, making corrections, and moving forward with resolve.

- **Honesty**: Many people fall into the trap of lying to themselves about their progress, effort, or commitment level. John, Tim, and Emilio each discovered the hard way that ignoring reality only prolongs the struggle. Honesty isn't just about admitting your current habits aren't working—it's about accepting that you're capable of change and growth. The sooner you stop the self-deception, the sooner you start making real gains.

- **Patience Over Quick Fixes**: The results worth having don't come fast, and trying to rush the process often leads to frustration or burnout. Tim's story, in particular, emphasized the cost of waiting until it's too late and expecting an instant turnaround. Developing patience is recognizing that sustainable change takes time, but each day you stick to the plan, you're building the foundation for lasting results.

- **Commitment to Consistency**: Consistency is your backbone—whether it's in the gym, the kitchen, or the small, daily habits that support your goals. Emilio's story is a testament to this. He saw real progress only when he stuck to a plan without getting distracted by fads. Commitment means showing up, even when you don't feel like it, because consistency compounds over time and brings results.

- **Avoiding Perfectionism**: Many people expect their journey to be flawless, but the truth is, setbacks are inevitable. Instead of letting one bad day ruin your motivation, learn to view setbacks as part of the process. You don't have to be perfect; you just have to be persistent. Allow yourself room to stumble, as long as you keep moving forward.

- **Self-Compassion**: Embracing a no-BS approach doesn't mean being harsh on yourself. Real change happens when you balance honesty with compassion, recognizing both your effort and your need to keep pushing forward. Self-compassion helps you sustain the journey without burning out or becoming overly critical.

Real Results: Lessons from Real People

The case studies in this book—John, Tim, and Emilio—weren't chosen randomly. Each of their stories illustrates a different path, different obstacles, and ultimately, different forms of success. Here's a quick recap of what you can take from their journeys:

- **John's Story**: A regular gym-goer stuck in place, John was "doing the work" but without intensity or awareness of his habits. His journey showed that just "showing up" isn't enough; intentionality and self-awareness are essential. Once he took responsibility for his diet and started tracking, he saw changes he never imagined. His story is a reminder that getting real results requires you to do more than go through the motions—you have to own the process.

- **Tim's Story**: Tim waited until a heart attack forced him to take action. His story is a stark reminder that health shouldn't be taken for granted, and a reactive approach to fitness comes at a cost. His journey emphasizes the importance of preventative action and consistency, especially if you've put off taking care of yourself for too long. Don't wait for a wake-up call—get ahead of it.

- **Emilio's Story**: Emilio's journey was about reshaping a body that he had never seen as "fit." He realized he was stuck in the "skinny fat" zone, but it wasn't until he committed to a specific strength-training plan and personalized nutrition that he saw the results he wanted. His story teaches us that achieving body composition goals requires dedication to both a clear plan and the patience to see it through.

These transformations weren't about overnight fixes; they were about sustainable, hard-won progress. Each person faced different challenges, but they had one common denominator: they stopped lying to themselves. They took ownership of their habits, prioritized health, and found real change through real commitment.

The Importance of Personalization: Your Journey, Your Rules

If there's one constant in fitness, it's that no single path works for everyone. The same strategy that worked for John might not work for Tim or Emilio, and that's because each journey is unique. There is no "one-size-fits-all" approach here; real results come from a plan that works for *you* and aligns with *your* goals, lifestyle, and preferences.

Personalization isn't about trying every trend out there; it's about testing, adapting, and creating a process you can stick with. When you tailor your journey to your own needs, you stop chasing fads and start creating results that last.

In summary, the path to your goals is built on core principles—tracking, portion control, and mindset shifts—and the understanding that your journey is entirely your own. Learn from the experiences in this book, but remember that your success comes from creating a sustainable, personal approach. You're in control, and with these tools, you're more than equipped to achieve the results you want.

TL;DR

This isn't a magic solution; it's a fucking call to action. If you think you can just skim the TL;DR and skip the work, you're mistaken. Real weight loss demands commitment and effort. You have to actively track your calories, move your ass, manage your portions, and cultivate the right mindset. No shortcuts—just hard work and real results. Now get out there and own it!

Core Principles of Real Weight Loss:

1. **Calorie Tracking:**

   - Use apps like MyFitnessPal or Lose It! to monitor your food intake.
   - Set and adjust your daily calorie targets based on your goals and progress. Log your meals and track your macros consistently.

2. **Physical Activity:**

   - Get moving! If the gym isn't your thing, find alternatives like walking, running, or any activity you enjoy. Check out the workout plans in the book for guidance.

3. **Master Portion Control:**

   - Pay attention to your hunger cues and practice mindful eating. Aim for a balanced plate: half vegetables, a quarter protein, and a quarter carbohydrates. Use visual cues and meal prep to manage portions effectively.

4. **Mindset Shifts:**

   - **Accountability:** Take responsibility for your habits and choices.
   - **Honesty:** Acknowledge where you are and commit to making changes.
   - **Patience:** Understand that real change takes time.
   - **Consistency:** Be committed to daily actions that support your goals.
   - **Self-Compassion:** Be honest with yourself, but also practice kindness.

The Power of Consistency

Consistency as a Key Ingredient

If you've read this far, you're already aware that there's no shortcut to achieving lasting weight loss. But even after laying down your goals, creating a plan, and getting all the right tools in place, it's the day-in, day-out effort that makes the magic happen. Consistency isn't about perfection; it's about building momentum with small, steady steps.

Think about it this way: a single workout won't make a visible change, just like one healthy meal won't instantly transform your body. But stick to that pattern—show up to the gym even when you don't feel like it, make smart food choices day after day, and those small efforts compound. Consistency separates the results-driven from the rest, and it's the defining factor behind real, lasting change.

Here's the truth: You don't need to have perfect days, just enough days where you did more right than wrong. That's the beauty of consistency—it's a commitment to keep showing up, rain or shine, win or lose. You don't need to go big every time; you just need to go.

Building Habits: Make Consistency Stick

Creating a consistent routine starts with building habits that feel natural and automatic over time. It may sound daunting, but you don't have to flip your whole life upside down in one go. Start small, lock in each habit one by one, and before you know it, those habits will become second nature. Here are some no-BS ways to build the foundation of consistency through habits:

Start Small

Going all in from day one sounds ambitious, but it's a recipe for burnout. The secret is to start with small, manageable goals. Try adding five minutes to your workout each day, or focus on hitting a single nutritional target like adding more protein to each meal. This "micro-habit" approach gives you easy wins and sets up a steady foundation to build on.

Use Triggers to Reinforce Habits

A "trigger" is something that reminds you to do a specific behavior. For example, brushing your teeth could be a trigger to drink a glass of water right after. Or maybe you'll use the moment you get home from work as a trigger to get into workout clothes right away. Setting up cues like this helps train your brain to associate a daily routine with a healthy habit. You don't need a long list; just start with one or two triggers and see how they boost your consistency.

Reward Yourself for Small Wins!

Celebrate the small wins along the way—it's not all about reaching the final goal. Recognizing progress keeps you motivated, so take a moment to acknowledge each little step forward. Just remember, rewarding yourself doesn't mean a huge splurge; maybe it's a break, a hobby you enjoy, or just the satisfaction of knowing you're one step closer. The goal is to make consistency feel positive, so you'll want to keep going.

Dealing with Setbacks: Embrace the Bumps

Let's get real: setbacks will happen. There's no way around it, no matter how much motivation or planning you have. Maybe it's a busy week, an injury, a vacation, or just one of those days where nothing goes right. Whatever the reason, setbacks are a given—not a signal to quit.

Expect, Don't Dread

The sooner you accept that setbacks are part of the journey, the better off you'll be. Going into your weight loss journey with the mindset that some days will be tough prepares you for them. A rough day doesn't undo your progress; it's just one moment on a much longer road. The key is to accept setbacks without letting them throw you off course.

Shift Your Perspective

Think of setbacks as learning moments instead of failures. Maybe you skipped a workout because you were tired; that's a chance to look at your sleep schedule. Or if you had a high-calorie weekend, use it as an opportunity to re-evaluate your planning and see where you could have made different choices. Learn, adjust, and keep moving.

Plan Ahead for Roadblocks

Life doesn't pause for your goals. Holidays, social events, stressful weeks—they're all going to test your consistency. Instead of hoping they won't disrupt your routine, go in with a plan:

- **Travel or Holidays**: Stick to basics by focusing on portion control, protein, and water intake. When it's harder to count calories or hit the gym, these small actions still help.
- **Busy Weeks**: Prep your meals in advance, even if they're simple, and keep your workouts short but intense. Even a quick workout is better than none.

- **Stressful Days**: Have a stress-relief plan that doesn't involve food—go for a walk, listen to music, or practice breathing exercises.

The aim is to stay consistent enough to maintain progress, even if things aren't perfect.

Consistency may not be glamorous, but it's your strongest ally in achieving results. You're building more than just a new routine; you're building resilience, discipline, and the confidence that comes from sticking to a plan. Embrace each step, learn from the setbacks, and remember: every small action is bringing you closer to real, lasting change.

Get fired up and go for it!

Ignite Your Passion for Change!

Listen up: you didn't pick up this book just to read. You're here because you want to get real results, and that means it's time to stop half-assing it. The truth is, this journey is going to be tough—there'll be days when you want to quit, days when it feels like nothing's working. But here's the deal: **you don't get results by giving up.** You get results by **showing the hell up** even when it's hard, even when you're tired, even when every part of you is screaming to sit back and coast. You didn't come this far just to turn around now.

You've got everything you need to smash your goals, but you have to use it. **I've handed you the shovel—now dig that damn hole!** Blast the laziness in the head with it if you have to. Stop waiting for some perfect moment or magical motivation to hit you—it's not coming. What's coming is a version of you that doesn't give up, that keeps grinding, that gets up, pushes harder, and goes for it even when everyone else would've quit.

Step Up and Take Action!

So here's the challenge: **stop making excuses, and start making progress.** Take one real, committed action today, right now. Plan out that workout. Track what you eat. Set a weekly goal and **fucking stick to it**. The little steps you take today are the ones that will push you over the line tomorrow.

This journey belongs to you. Own it with everything you've got. There's no holding back, no cutting corners, no waiting around. You're not just reading about change—you're making it happen. So get out there, crush it, and don't stop until you're proud. **Go make your damn goals a reality.**

Final Thoughts

Reiterate Commitment

As you reach the end of this journey, remember this: **commitment is the bedrock of all progress.** You've taken the first step by picking up this book, but the real work lies ahead. True transformation demands dedication, grit, and the relentless pursuit of your goals. Embrace the struggles and celebrate the victories, no matter how small.

Every workout, every meal, every choice adds up. **Understand that setbacks are not failures; they are opportunities to learn and grow.** You're not just building a physique—you're building a mindset. Every drop of sweat and every ounce of effort you put forth is a step closer to the person you aspire to be. **Stay committed—your future self will thank you!**

So, as you step forward, carry this mantra with you: **"I will not back down. I will not quit. I will push through."** Let this commitment fuel your fire and propel you toward the greatness that awaits.

Invitation for Feedback

I want to hear from you! **Your experiences, challenges, and triumphs matter.** Whether you crushed your goals or faced setbacks, sharing your journey can inspire others and create a powerful community of support.

Don't keep your story to yourself! Reach out—send me your thoughts, share your progress, and let's build this movement together. Your voice can be the spark that ignites someone else's motivation. We're all in this fight for real results, and together, we'll make it happen!

Closing Statement

You hold the key to your transformation! This journey isn't just about losing weight or building muscle; it's about reclaiming your life and embracing your true potential. Each page you've turned has led you to this moment, and now it's time to take action.

Remember, success isn't a destination; it's a relentless pursuit fueled by commitment, hard work, and unwavering belief in yourself. **The path ahead may be challenging, but every step you take brings you closer to the life you've envisioned.**

So rise up! Shake off the doubts, drown out the negativity, and step boldly into your future. **You are capable of greatness, and the world is waiting to see what you can achieve.** Take these lessons to heart, trust the process, and never lose sight of your goals.

This is not the end; it's just the beginning. **Go forth and conquer!** Your journey is yours to own, and with each passing day, you're one step closer to becoming the person you were always meant to be.

Now get the fuck out there and make it happen!

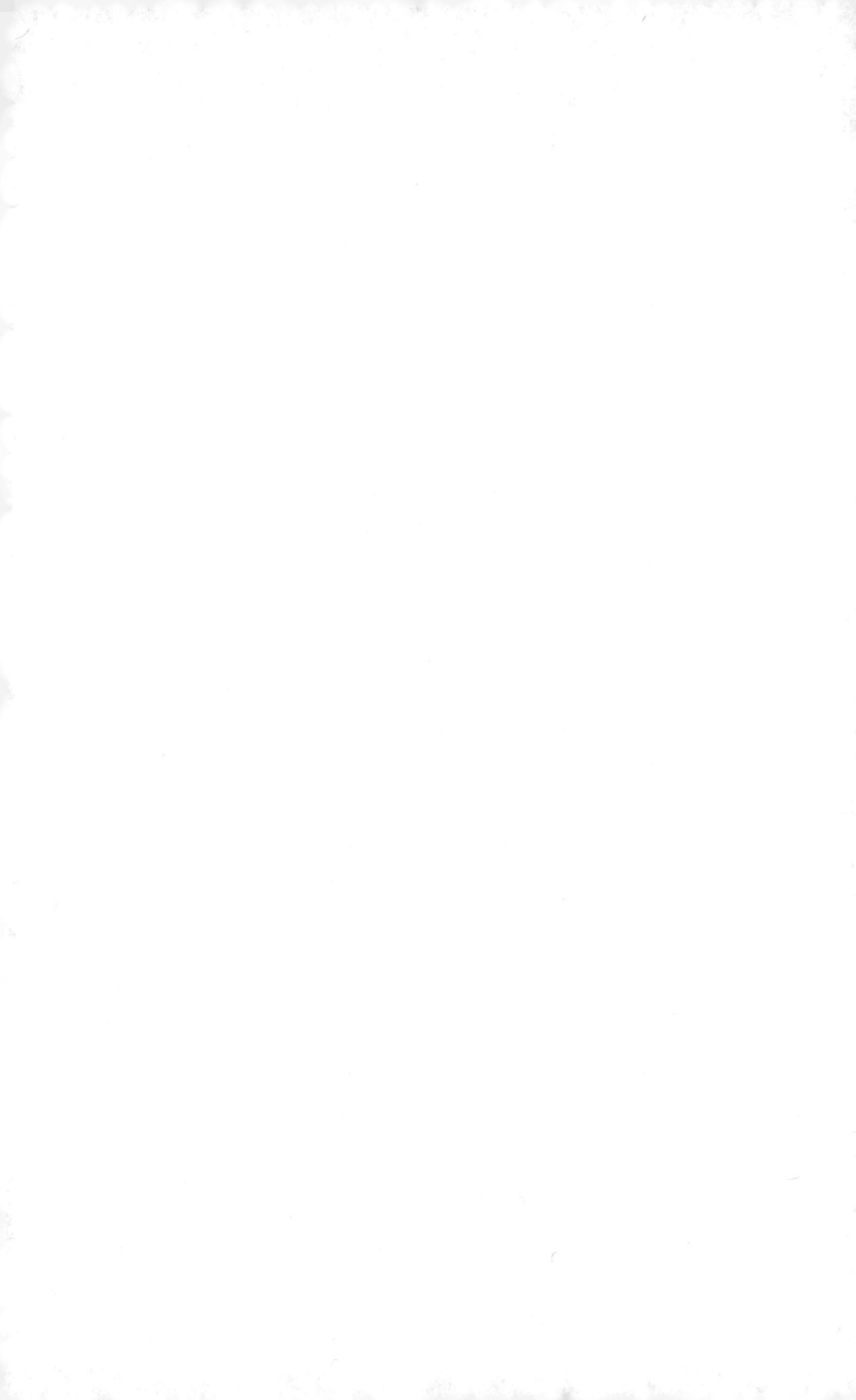